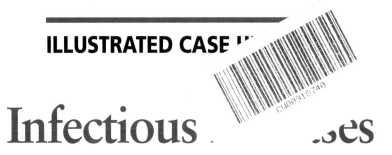

ILLUSTRATED CASE H...

Infectious ......es

Nick J. Beeching, MA BM BCh MRCP FRACP DCH DTM&H

Senior Lecturer in Infectious Diseases
Liverpool School of Tropical Medicine
Liverpool, UK

Honorary Consultant Physician
Regional Infectious Disease Unit
Fazakerley Hospital
Liverpool, UK

John S. Cheesbrough, BSc MB BS MRCP MRCPath

Consultant Microbiologist
Blackburn Royal Infirmary
Blackburn, UK

Honorary Research Fellow
University Department of Medical Microbiology
    and Genitourinary Medicine
The University of Liverpool
Liverpool, UK

WITH COMPLIMENTS

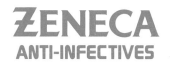

Copyright © 1994 Mosby–Year Book Europe Limited
Published in 1994 by Wolfe Publishing, an imprint of Mosby–Year Book
Europe Limited

Printed by BPCC Hazell Books Ltd, Aylesbury, England

ISBN 0 7234 1799 7

    For full details of all Mosby–Year Book Europe Limited titles please write
to Mosby–Year Book Europe Limited, Lynton House, 7–12 Tavistock, Square,
London WC1H 9LB, England.

A CIP catalogue record for this book is available from the British Library.

Library of Congress Cataloging-in-Publication Data has been applied for

---

Warning

The doses of pharmaceutical products given in this book are a guide only. Although
every effort is made to be accurate, the authors and publishers cannot be held
responsible for the accuracy of these dosages. It is recommended that the reader,
if in any doubt, checks in the latest editions of publications such as the British
National Formulary, Martindale's Extra Pharmacopoeia or MIMS (Monthly Index of
Medical Specialities).

Contents

Preface

The aim of this book is to provide illustrative cases that will be of relevance to all who have an interest in infectious disease practice in its widest sense. The diagnostic approaches to the problems presented range from the purely 'clinical' to the predominantly laboratory oriented, but the majority of cases have been chosen to emphasise the interaction between these complementary disciplines. Although we have included some of the major imported infections, the range of cases has been selected to show that infectious disease practice is no longer confined to traditional fever hospital medicine. Many of the patients initially presented to medical or surgical teams and continued to be managed on general hospital wards or in intensive care units. However, we do not pretend to have covered the whole of infectious disease or clinical microbiological practice, but we have attempted to illustrate as wide a range of diagnostic methodologies as possible.

Each case history is presented as a challenge for the reader to formulate his or her own diagnostic and management plan, with the answers immediately following. We have been didactic where appropriate, but local practice varies enormously with geographical differences in the prevalence of pathogens and their sensitivity to antimicrobials, local or national prescribing policies and mere fashion. The case histories are suitable for postgraduate students to read alone or for discussion in group tutorials. We anticipate that one of the major challenges in either situation will be to identify areas in which local practice differs from our own answers, and to identify the reasons for this. We have tried to highlight the main points relevant to each case, and hope that these will stimulate the reader to enquire after further detail in more comprehensive textbooks or current journals.

In order to simplify the case histories, the majority of the common haematological and biochemical investigations have been abbreviated and presented in a stylised format. Abbreviations, normal ranges in SI units and conversion factors are summarised on page 7. Where relevant, we have emphasised the importance of community control of infections, including timely notification. In Britain the term 'public health authorities' in the text means the local consultant in public health medicine or consultant in communicable disease control. We have used the more generic term in recognition that the appropriate statutory authority will vary in other countries.

Nick Beeching
John Cheesbrough

Acknowledgements

Above all others, we thank our families for tolerating prolonged disruption of normal social life while we were collating these case histories. We also thank our many previous teachers, mentors and colleagues who have allowed us to use cases or material (see list below) and particularly thank Dr Fred Nye and Professor Tony Hart for their continued support, encouragement and suggestions.

For general assistance with photography we acknowledge the Departments of Medical Illustration of the Aintree Hospitals NHS Trust, Auckland Hospital, Blackburn Royal Infirmary, Birmingham Heartlands Hospital, the Liverpool School of Tropical Medicine and the Royal Liverpool University Hospital. Specific extra photography for the book was performed by Noel Blundell, Debbie Sutherland and Brian Getty of the Department of Medical Microbiology and Genitourinary Medicine, Royal Liverpool University Hospital, and Graham Watson of the Department of Medical Illustration of the Liverpool School of Tropical Medicine. We also thank Drs Bill Taylor and Peter Southall for performing autopsies on our HIV-positive patients at Fazakerley Hospital and for providing many of the histopathological slides.

Miss Jean Taylor has patiently converted our heiroglyphs into a coherent manuscript and we thank her for her customary dependability and efficiency. Finally, we are grateful to our publishers for their unflagging support, particularly Geoff Greenwood and subsequently Maire Collins.

The cases presented in this book have been seen by us over the past 10 years. As far as we are aware, few of the clinical photographs have been published before and these are specifically acknowledged below. We apologise if there are any inadvertent omissions from this list or the following alphabetical list of colleagues who have contributed material or provided useful comments:

Dr KD Allen
Mrs JW Bailey
Mr A Bakran
Dr DR Bell
Dr PMA Calverley
Prof CJ Cawley
Dr IM Chesner
Dr AB Christie
Dr RE Clark
Dr BM Daly
Dr J Danher
Dr PDO Davies
Dr CJ Edwards
Dr RB Ellis-Pegler
Dr BF Eyes
Dr ID Farrell
Prof RG Finch
Dr R Fox
Dr NJ French
Prof AM Geddes

Dr IT Gilmore
Mr MW Guy
Dr N Hardwick
Prof CA Hart
Dr CRM Hay
Dr T Helliwell
Dr M Jones
Dr SDR Lang
Mrs B Lee
Dr A List
Dr JM MacKenzie
Mr T Makin
Dr JC McGregor
Dr ME Molyneux
Dr KJ Mutton
Dr FJ Nye
Dr CJ Parry
Dr JR Playfer

Dr AE Prevost
Dr JD Rhodes
Ms K Robotham
Dr S Saltissi
Mr RA Sells
Mr IM Shaw
Dr DH Smith
Dr GW Smith
Mr A Soorae
Dr PJ Southall
Dr W Taylor
Dr CYW Tong
Mr SA Walkinshaw
Dr DC Warhurst
Dr RG Wilkes
Prof JC Woodrow
Mr A Wu
Dr GB Wyatt

Other publishers

Figures **1** and **3** in Case 26 are reproduced by kind permission of authors and publishers from page 24 of *A Colour Atlas of Respiratory Infections* by Macfarlane, JT., Finch, RG., Cotton, RE., Chapman & Hall Medical, London, 1993.

Normal adult values and abbreviations

	SI Units	Alternatives	Approximate numerical conversion (SI to alternative)
Haematology			
Haemoglobin (Hb)	Male 14–18 g/dl Female 12–16 g/dl	mg/100 ml mg/100 ml	Same Same
Haematocrit (Hct)	Male 0.42–0.52 Female 0.37–0.47	% %	×100 ×100
Mean cell volume (MCV)	77–98 fl	Same	
Peripheral white blood cell count(WBC)	$4–10 \times 10^9/l$	$4,000–10,000/mm^3$	×1000
Platelets	$150–450 \times 10^9/l$	$150,000–450,000/mm^3$	×1000
Prothrombin time	≤14 sec		Same
Prothrombin ratio (INR)	≤1.2		Same
Partial thromboplastin time (APTT)	28–30 sec		Same
Erythrocyte sedimentation rate (ESR)	<15 mm/hr		Same
C-reactive protein	<10 mg/l	<10 ng/ml	Same
Serum biochemistry			
Sodium (Na)	136–144 mmol/l	mEq/l	Same
Potassium (K)	3.5–5.0 mmol/l	mEq/l	Same
Urea	2.5–7.5 mmol/l	15–45 mg/100 ml	×6
Creatinine	0–110 μmol/l	0–1.2 mg/100 ml	Divide by 100
Glucose (fasting)	3.6–5.8 mmol/l	65–105 mg/100 ml	×18
Bilirubin total	0–22 μmol/l	0–1.2 mg %	Divide by 18
Aspartate transaminase (AST)	5–45 u/l	(SGOT)	Same

	SI Units	Alternatives	Approximate numerical conversion (SI to alternative)
Serum biochemistry *(continued)*			
Alanine transaminase (ALT)	5–45 u/l	(SGPT)	Same
Gamma-glutamyl transferase (γGT)	0–30 u/l	(GGT)	Same
Alkaline phosphatase (alk. phos.)	30–130 u/l	Several	Varies
Albumin	36–50 g/l	3.6–5.0 g/100 ml	Divide by 10
Total protein	60–80 g/l	6.0–8.0 g/100 ml	Divide by 10
Arterial blood gases (breathing room air)			
pH	7.36–7.45		Same
Base excess (BE)	-2.5– +2.5 mmol/l	mEq/l	Same
Standard bicarbonate (standard HCO_3)	22–26 mmol/l	mEq/l	Same
Oxygen tension (pO_2)	12–15 kPa	90–112 mmHg	×7.5
Carbon dioxide tension (pCO_2)	4.5–6.1 kPa	34–46 mmHg	×7.5
Cerebrospinal fluid (CSF)			
Pressure	8–18 cm H_2O		Same
White blood cells (WBC)	$<5 \times 10^6$/l	$<5/mm^3$	Same
Red blood cells (RBC)	$<1 \times 10^6$/l	$<1/mm^3$	Same
Total protein	<0.45 g/l	<45 mg/100 ml	×100
Glucose	3.5–4.5 mmol/l	63–80 mg %	×18
CSF glucose: blood glucose ratio	>0.4		

Other abbreviations

AFB	acid fast bacillus
AIDS	acquired immune deficiency syndrome
ARDS	adult respiratory distress syndrome
BAL	bronchoalveolar lavage
bid	twice daily
BP	blood pressure
CCDC	Consultant in Communicable Disease Control
CD4+cells	CD4 antigen-bearing T lymphocytes (OKT4 cells, T-helper cells)
CFT	complement fixation test
CK	creatinine kinase
CMV	cytomegalovirus infection
CNS	central nervous system
CT	computed tomography
DIC	disseminated intravascular coagulation
DNA	deoxyribonucleic acid
ELISA	enzyme linked immunosorbent assay
FAT	fluorescent antibody test
HIV	human immunodeficiency virus
IFAT	indirect fluorescent antibody test
ITU	intensive care unit
IV	intravenous
IVU	intravenous urogram
LFTs	liver function tests
MAC	*Mycobacterium avium* complex
MBC	minimum bactericidal concentration (of antimicrobial)
MIC	minimum inhibitory concentration (of antimicrobial)
MR	magnetic resonance (imaging)
MSSU	mid-stream specimen of urine
PCP	*Pneumocystis carinii* pneumonia
PCR	polymerase chain reaction
PUO	pyrexia of unknown origin
qid	four times a day
RIBA	recombinant immunoblot assay
SLE	systemic lupus erythematosus
TB	tuberculosis
tid	three times a day
TPHA	*Treponema pallidum* haemagglutination assay
VDRL	Venereal Disease Reference Laboratory test for syphilis
WHO	World Health Organization
ZN	Ziehl–Neelsen stain

Case 1

Pulmonary problem in renal transplant recipient

History

A 66-year-old woman is admitted to hospital with a 2-week history of non-productive cough associated with pleuritic chest pain and which has failed to respond to a 7-day course of Augmentin® (co-amoxyclav).

She has a history of renal failure due to chronic pyelonephritis with associated hypertension and has required haemodialysis for the last 3 years. A pacemaker had been implanted a year ago for episodes of bradycardia attributed to ischaemic heart disease. Six weeks prior to admission she had received a cadaveric renal transplant. Two episodes of rejection responded to pulsed high-dose methylprednisolone and she is currently receiving oral cyclosporin A and prednisolone.

On examination her temperature is 38.5°C and her respiratory rate is 19. Her chest is clear and there is no tenderness over the renal graft or pacemaker unit. No other abnormalities are found in any system.

Haematology:	Hb 11.2 g/dl WBC 7.8 × 10⁹/l Neutrophils 70%, lymphocytes 25%, monocytes 3% Platelets 200 × 10⁹/l
Biochemistry:	Na 137 mmol/l K 4.3 mmol/l Creatinine 179 µmol/l Liver function tests normal
Radiology:	Illustrated opposite (**1, 2**)
Serology:	Anti-cytomegalovirus complement fixation tests (anti-CMV CFTs) are illustrated opposite (**3**)

Questions

1 What abnormalities are present on the chest x-rays?
2 How would you interpret the CMV serology?
3 What pathogens would you consider as leading causes of her pulmonary disease?
4 What further investigations would you perform?
5 What additional points in the history would you ask about?

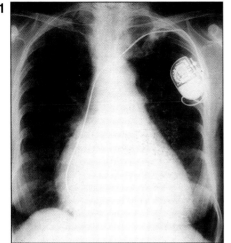 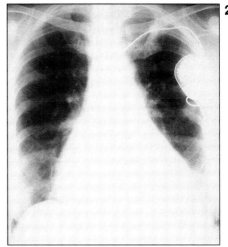

1 Chest x-ray prior to renal transplant.   **2** Chest x-ray on admission.

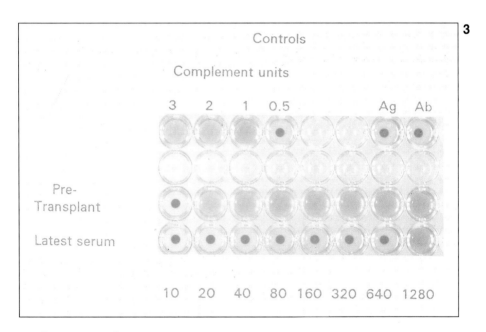

3 CFTs for anti-CMV antibodies (Ag = antigen; Ab = antibody).

Case 1

Answers

1   Both chest x-rays show a fibrotic calcified left apical lesion and moderate cardiomegaly. A new peripheral coin lesion has developed below the pacemaker unit (**2**).

2   The serology shows a rise in anti-CMV CFT from 1:10 at the time of transplant to 1:640. The marked rise in CMV antibody titre, which was present at low level prior to the transplant, indicates that reinfection from the grafted kidney or endogenous reactivation of CMV has occurred. This is common after renal transplantation and is not usually associated with serious disease. Reactivation of CMV is, however, associated with an increased risk of opportunistic infection. Primary CMV infection in an immunosuppressed patient is typically a more serious illness characterised by fever, bone marrow suppression and signs of gastrointestinal or diffuse pulmonary disease.

3   The apical lesion is strongly suggestive of previous tuberculosis. In the context of her immunosuppression, likely causes for the coin lesion are mycobacteria and *Nocardia* sp. Other opportunists, such as cyptococcus or aspergillus, are less likely but the possibility of a pyogenic abscess related to right-sided endocarditis secondary to the pacemaker wire might be considered. CMV or *Pneumocystis carinii* pneumonitis are unlikely to present with such a focal lesion. Histoplasmosis or coccidioidomycosis would be remote possibilities if there was an appropriate travel history.

4   Direct sampling of the lesion is essential and percutaneous aspiration or biopsy is the method of choice for such a peripheral lesion. This was undertaken and the Gram stain of the pus obtained shows branching Gram-positive bacilli compatible with either nocardia or actinomyces (**4**). These possibilities can be rapidly distinguished by Ziehl–Neelsen stain using weak (2%) sulphuric acid to decolourise the stain (**5**). *Nocardia* sp. retain the stain; they grow aerobically (**6**) and are resistant to penicillin, which again contrasts with the anaerobic, penicillin-sensitive actinomyces. Differentiation of the major species of nocardia, *N. asteroides* and *N. brasiliensis*, relies on biochemical tests which are best performed in a reference laboratory.

Clinically important points to remember about nocardial infection are:

- The frequency with which metastatic infection may occur. Brain abscess occurs in approximately 25% of all cases and other common sites include liver and skin.
- The coexistence of other opportunist infections, particularly *P. carinii* and *Mycobacterium tuberculosis.*
- The limited relevance of *in vitro* sensitivity testing. This usually reveals sensitivity to sulphonamides, erythromycin, amikacin (but not other aminoglycosides) and imipenem. However, the only agents with which there is extensive clinical experience are sulphonamides in high doses and co-trimoxazole. Sulphonamides have effected cures in the face of *in vitro* resistance and should be regarded as the agents of first choice. A high dose, typically 6 g of sulphamethoxazole/day, is necessary, but this will require modification in patients with renal impairment in whom blood levels should be checked. Treatment should be prolonged and 6 weeks would usually be regarded as the minimum.

4 Pus aspirated from peripheral coin lesion. Gram stain showing branching Gram-positive bacilli.

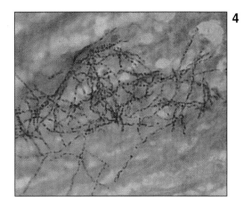

4

5 Modified Ziehl–Neelsen stain of Nocardia asteroides.

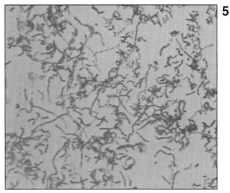

5

6 Pigmented mucoid colonies of N. asteroides after 5 days of aerobic culture on blood agar.

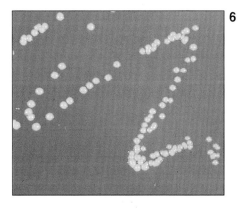

6

5   It is essential to discover if she has ever suffered from tuberculosis, and if she has travelled in the tropics or the USA. If she has never received any chemotherapy for TB, she is at high risk of recrudescence now. Patients entering dialysis programmes are at relatively high risk of reactivation of previous TB and those with evidence of past TB should receive prophylaxis with isoniazid for 9 months or rifampicin with isoniazid for 6 months. The risk is even greater after transplantation, and any patients previously overlooked should be treated similarly at that stage.

Case 1

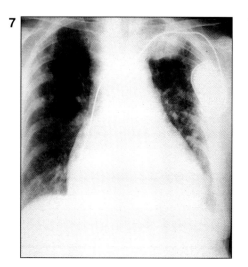

7 Chest x-ray shortly prior to death.

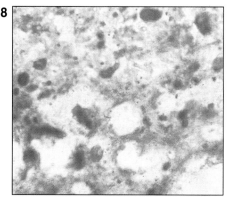
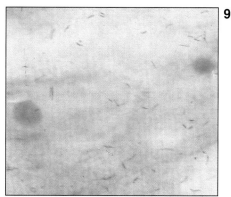

8, 9 Abscess material obtained at autopsy showing mycobacterial 'ghosts' on Gram stain (**8**) and acid-fast bacilli on Ziehl–Neelsen stain (**9**).

Progress

She received co-trimoxazole in high doses and initially responded with a fall in her temperature. The dosage was reduced as her renal function deteriorated and fever recurred after 10 days' treatment. Her general condition then deteriorated and a repeat chest x-ray (**7**) showed expansion of the apical lesion and widespread nodular infiltrates. Antituberculous treatment was started but she died 3 days later. At autopsy a large tuberculous abscess of the caecum and mesenteric lymph nodes was found, with a smaller abscess at the apex of the left lung. Histology of the lung showed widespread poorly defined granulomata containing numerous acid-fast bacilli and *M. tuberculosis* was cultured from lung and mesentery (**8**, **9**).

Case 2

The eyes have it

History

A 45-year-old man presents with a 2-week history of soreness of both eyes and pains in the hands and lower legs. He admits to having had general malaise, a congested nose and a vague fever for almost a month, but is not very forthcoming about other symptoms or his past medical history. He comes from a poor family and has lived all his life in the Middle East.

Examination shows an unwell-looking man with a temperature of 37.8°C, a pulse of 90 and blood pressure of 120/75. His facial appearance is shown in **1**. His skin feels slightly thickened and there is bilateral pretibial oedema. There is painful warmth, swelling and tenderness of the left ankle and over several interphalangeal joints of the fingers (**2**). There are no focal cardiac, respiratory or neurological signs, and there is no thyroid enlargement.

Haematology:	Hb 11.5 g/dl
	WBC 15.6 × 10⁹/l
	Neutrophils 80%, lymphocytes 15%
	Platelets 400 × 10⁹/L
	ESR 103 mm/hr
Biochemistry:	Urea and electrolytes normal
	Liver function tests normal
	Albumin 38 g/l, total protein 80 g/l
Radiology:	Chest x-ray normal
Serology:	Screen for rheumatoid factor positive
	VDRL positive, TPHA negative

Questions

1 What physical signs are present?
2 What is the differential diagnosis?
3 How would you investigate his condition?
4 How would you manage this patient?

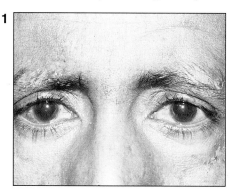

1 Face of patient.

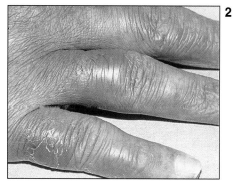

2 Swollen lesions on fingers.

Case 2

Answers

1   There are nodular infiltrated lesions in the eyebrows with associated loss of hair. There is perilimbal erythema of both conjunctivae, more pronounced on the right, suggesting uveitis.

2   The combination of polyarthritis and uveitis suggests a seronegative arthritis including Reiter's syndrome, systemic lupus erythematosus (SLE), sarcoidosis, or an immune complex disease. Sarcoidosis is unlikely in a patient from this region and Reiter's syndrome does not usually involve the fingers or cause the skin lesions shown. While these findings and the serological results are compatible with SLE, any rash or obscure rheumatological problem in a patient who has lived in the tropics should raise the possibility of leprosy. Patients with lepromatous leprosy may have very subtle skin changes without gross neurological deficit. The acute presentation with features of immune complex disease and pretibial oedema is that of the lepra reaction (erythema nodosum leprosum, ENL). Erythema nodosum is not always obvious in this reactional state and is not restricted to the limbs (3–5).

Nerve involvement is diffuse in multibacillary leprosy and may be difficult to detect. There was no palpable enlargement of the supraorbital nerves in the patient illustrated. More obvious nerve involvement, with sensory and motor deficits and nerve thickening, occurs in paucibacillary leprosy. Diabetes does not cause nerve thickening, which should always be excluded in a diabetic who has lived in the tropics and has peripheral neuropathy.

3   The results of the investigations already performed are all compatible with the clinical diagnosis, revealing neutrophilia, a high ESR, raised globulins due to high levels of IgG, false-positive rheumatoid latex test and false-positive reagin test. Specific diagnosis is made by Ziehl–Neelsen (6), or auramine-phenol stains of swabs or nose-blow specimens of nasal secretions and by examination of slit-skin smears taken from several sites of the body. In the absence of identifiable areas of abnormal skin these are conventionally taken from the earlobes, the back, and the dorsum of the fingers. Skin biopsy shows infiltration with large numbers of acid-fast bacilli within foamy macrophages (7).

4   Specific chemotherapy should be instituted according to 1982 WHO guidelines for treatment of multibacillary leprosy and so he was initially given, daily, rifampicin 600 mg, dapsone 100 mg and clofazimine 50 mg. This was subsequently changed to clofazimine 50 mg and dapsone 100 mg both daily, supplemented by supervised doses of rifampicin 600 mg and clofazimine 300 mg at his monthly clinic visits. Therapy should be supervised by an expert and should continue for a minimum of 2 years. His reactional state was managed with bed rest and a rapidly reducing course of oral prednisolone starting with a dose of 40 mg daily. Clofazimine has anti-inflammatory activity and may prevent recurrence of reactions, which are common during the first year of chemotherapy. If these do occur, the dose of clofazimine can be increased. Carefully supervised thalidomide therapy may be necessary to manage reactional states, but this should never be given to women of childbearing age and male patients must be warned not to pass on their tablets to any other person. The public health authorities were notified of the patient's diagnosis, and his family contacts were reviewed for symptoms but none had evidence of infection.

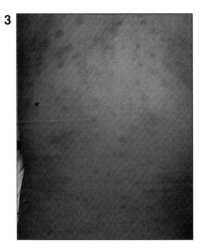

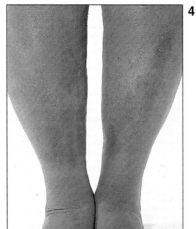

3 Multiple lesions of erythema nodosum leprosum (ENL) on back of a Pacific islander.

4 Acute lesions on legs of same patient as in Figure **3**. Lesions are stained by clofazimine.

5 Resolution of ENL in same patient 3 weeks later, with peeling skin and loss of oedema.

6 Large numbers of acid-fast bacilli in nasal smear (Ziehl–Neelsen stain).

7 Skin biopsy in lepromatous leprosy showing numerous acid-fast bacilli in vacuolated macrophages in dermis (Fite-Faraco stain).

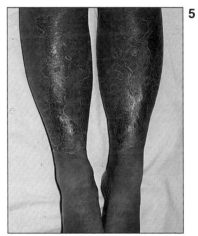

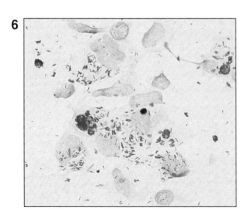

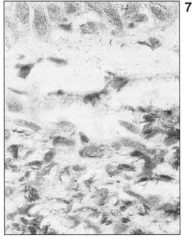

Collapse on a world tour

History

A 55-year-old French woman is brought to the emergency room of an Auckland hospital after collapsing at the international airport. She had never left France before until embarking on a world tour 6 weeks previously. She first went to Nairobi in Kenya for 4 days and spent 2 days on safari and a further 8 days at a beach hotel near Mombasa. Prior to departure she had a full course of immunisations – including one for yellow fever – and started taking regular amodiaquine chemoprophylaxis. Apart from mild diarrhoea for 24 hours shortly after arrival in Kenya, her health in Africa remained good. She then flew to the east coast of the USA to start a Greyhound tour across America. Two weeks after leaving Kenya she developed non-bloody diarrhoea up to 5 times a day and felt vaguely unwell with occasional fever and sweats. She stopped taking her amodiaquine but diarrhoea and malaise continued until she reached the west coast. She was unable to leave her hotel for 3 days due to continued diarrhoea and dizziness on standing but was ultimately able to catch her flight to New Zealand.

On direct questioning, her major complaints are of diarrhoea, an inability to sit up due to dizziness, and of bruises which have appeared on her abdomen over the past few days. She is unable to give any further history but does not appear to have any significant past medical history apart from mild asthma. Examination reveals an unwell woman with a clammy, pale periphery, an axillary temperature of 35.6°C, pulse of 130 and a respiratory rate of 24. Systolic blood pressure is 60 mmHg by palpation when lying and is unrecordable when she sits up. She has bruises on her trunk (1), but no lymphadenopathy or hepato-splenomegaly. Apart from drowsiness and intermittent confusion, there are no focal neurological signs. She is moved immediately to the intensive care unit (ITU) for further management (2).

Questions

1 What are the most likely diagnoses?
2 What is the relevance of the timing of her symptoms?
3 What are the other critical early investigations?
4 How would you manage her initially?

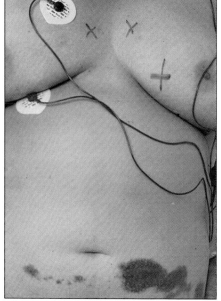

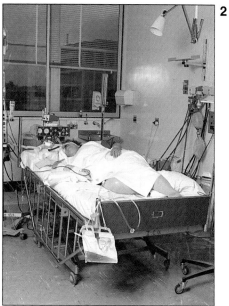

1   Bruising on admission.   2   Early management in ITU.

Initial investigations available in emergency room

Urine:	Protein +++, blood ++, urobilinogen +++
Haematology:	Hb 10.2 g/dl WBC 3×10^9/l Platelets 10×10^9/l
Biochemistry:	Na 128 mmol/l K 3.2 mmol/l Urea 18 mmol/l Creatinine 350 μmol/l Glucose 3.0 mmol/l
Arterial blood gases: (room air)	pH 7.25, base excess -25 mmol/l, pCO_2 3 kPa (23 mmHg) pO_2 10.4 kPa (78 mmHg)

Case 3

Answers

1 Malaria must always be considered when an ill traveller returns from a malaria endemic area, even if she has been taking regular chemoprophylaxis. Although the history is not 'typical' of malaria, diarrhoea is not infrequently a prominent symptom of expatriates with falciparum malaria. Fever may be absent at presentation and in this case was artefactually low because a peripheral temperature was taken in the presence of poor peripheral circulation. Many of her symptoms could be due to dehydration secondary to gastroenteritis of any origin, but the progressive diarrhoea and recent bruising raise the possibility of a salmonella infection (including typhoid) with septicaemia and disseminated intravascular coagulation (DIC). At this stage of typhoid infection, ileal perforation should be considered. Gram-negative septicaemia associated with urinary infection is a strong possibility. Borreliosis may present with fever and DIC but is unlikely to cause profuse diarrhoea. Acute leukaemia should be considered, despite the absence of lymphadenopathy or splenomegaly.

2 Patients with a febrile illness that starts within 3 weeks of leaving rural Africa may have a viral haemorrhagic fever (VHF), suggested by diarrhoea and bruising in this case. However, the patient had had only limited travelling experience in rural areas, and VHFs have only been reported rarely in expatriates visiting Kenya. The timing of onset of her symptoms is appropriate for malaria, the appearance of which may be delayed, especially in patients taking chemoprophylaxis.

3 Malarial films: Positive for falciparum malaria (**3-5**)
  DIC screen: Fibrin degradation products >12 µg/ml (normal <3)
                       Prothrombin ratio (INR) 2.5; APTT 60 seconds
  Blood cultures: Sterile
  Liver function tests: AST 180 u/l; alk. phos. 200 u/l; bilirubin 120
                       µmol/l

4 Supportive treatment should include supplemental oxygen and vigorous infusion of plasma expanders. In this case, Swann–Ganz catheterisation shortly after admission to the ITU showed a low pulmonary artery wedge pressure and further plasma expanders were given to bring this to mid-normal. Within 6 hours she developed pulmonary oedema with a high pulmonary artery wedge pressure, suggestive of fluid overload rather than acute respiratory distress syndrome (wedge pressure is usually low). She required intubation and assisted ventilation for the next 5 days. Broad-spectrum cephalosporins were given immediately after blood cultures had been drawn. Results of malaria films were available within 30 minutes of arrival and she was given a loading dose of IV quinine 20 mg base/kg over 4 hours. Thereafter, she was maintained on IV quinine 10 mg/kg 8 hourly for 7 days. Parasite rates were monitored every 12 hours and fell progressively to 1% at 72 hours, but occasional abnormal ring forms could still be seen for a further 3 days. Her low serum glucose was easily corrected and monitored frequently but severe hypoglycaemia was not a problem. Renal output was maintained and serum biochemistry gradually returned to normal. Her platelet count did not rise above $150 \times 10^9/l$ until the 10th day of admission.

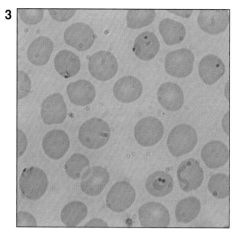
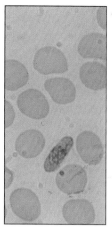

3, 4 Thin blood films showing 12% falciparum malaria parasitaemia with multiple ring forms (**3**) and gametocytes (**4**). Absolute parasite count 495 × 10⁹/l.

5 Thick blood film (Field's stain) showing numerous ring forms. The red cell structure is lost in the staining process.

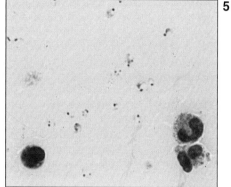

Recovery after extubation was uneventful apart from transient deafness and dizziness due to the quinine.

Clinically significant DIC rarely complicates malaria, although thrombocytopenia is common. It raises the possibility of concomitant Gram-negative sepsis, which is one possible cause of collapse in severe malaria. Other causes include hypoglycaemia and spontaneous rupture of the spleen (although this rare event is more typically associated with vivax malaria). The patient's pulmonary oedema was iatrogenic and might have been avoided by slightly less vigorous fluid replacement. She was lucky to survive, and her illness demonstrates that chemoprophylaxis does not always prevent malaria but rather may merely delay the onset of severe symptoms and protect against the lethal effects.

Amodiaquine, once commonly used by French travellers, has now been replaced by other regimens. Up-to-date advice on malaria chemoprophylaxis must be obtained if a trip to the tropics is planned, as drug-resistant malaria continues to spread throughout the world.

Case 4

The limping Samoan

History

A 56-year-old Western Samoan man attends the clinic with a 6-month history of back pain, worsening for 1 month with radiation to the abdomen and mild discomfort while walking. He has recently been troubled by general malaise, rigors, weight loss, hiccups, cough and constipation, and has been unable to smoke his usual 20 cigarettes a day due to altered taste sensation. He usually works on a plantation in Samoa and the only history of note is a prolonged episode of back pain and fever 3 years ago, for which he did not receive any treatment. He drinks '2 to 3' bottles of beer daily.

Examination shows an ill man with jaundice and a temperature of 39.2°C, pulse of 100 and blood pressure of 120/60. There are no signs of chronic liver disease, endocarditis or focal chest pathology. He is tender in the lower back, with bilaterally swollen paravertebral muscles (1). Bilateral masses are palpable deep in the abdomen. His liver is of normal size and is not tender. He is able to walk, with no localising neurological signs in the legs, but he experiences mild abdominal pain when his hips are hyperextended. Admission blood tests show:

Haematology:	Hb 12.9 g/dl
	WBC 21.8 × 10⁹/l
	Neutrophils 94% with left shift
	Platelets 567 × 10⁹/l
	ESR 143 mm/hr
Biochemistry:	Na 126 mmol/l
	K 4.0 mmol/l
	Urea 6.0 mmol/l
	Albumin 27 g/l, total protein 75 g/l
	Bilirubin 85 μmol/l
	Alk. phos. 225 u/l
	AST 135 u/l
	γGT 195 u/l
	Prothrombin ratio (INR) 1.6
Urine:	WBC 15 × 10⁶/l
	RBC 0
	Occasional granular casts
	Sterile on routine culture
Imaging:	Illustrated opposite (2–4)

Questions

1 What further points in the history might be relevant?
2 What do Figures **2**, **3** and **4** show?
3 What is the diagnosis and what are the possible underlying causes and infecting organisms?
4 What further investigations would you perform?
5 How should he be managed?

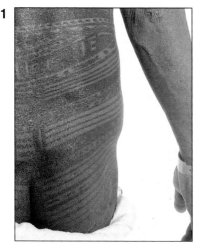

1 Prominent paravertebral muscles under traditional tattoos.

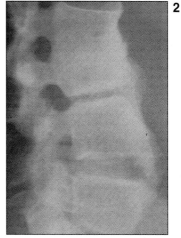

2 Lateral lumbar radiograph.

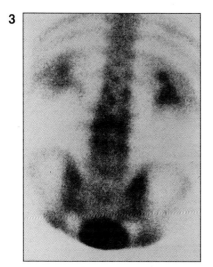

3 Technetium bone scan (posterior view).

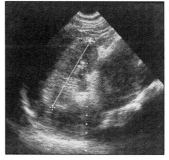

4 Sagittal ultrasound of abdomen (right kidney marked by measurement line).

Case 4

Answers

1 There was no personal or family history suggestive of tuberculosis. His impressive traditional tattoos had been done using ink and a sharpened stick in early adulthood, with no recent additions that might have introduced infection. There was no history of back injury and he did not abuse intravenous drugs.

2 Figure **2** shows loss of intervertebral disc L2/3 with partial collapse and fusion of the contiguous vertebrae, and anterior syndesmophytes down to L5 suggestive of old or chronic osteomyelitis. Figure **3** shows increased isotope uptake in L3 and L4. The ultrasound scan (**4**) shows a hyperechoic mass in the paravertebral region displacing the right kidney ventrally and cranially.

3 The diagnosis is bilateral psoas abscesses and chronic osteomyelitis. The most likely unifying diagnosis is staphylococcal osteomyelitis with forward extension into the psoas sheaths. This is supported by the positive 'femoral stretch test' described. Less stoical patients often have difficulty walking with such large abscesses. The liver function tests are compatible with consequences of septicaemia or with intrahepatic abscess. Tuberculosis is the most important alternative diagnosis. Psoas abscesses arising from bowel affected by diverticular disease, neoplasm or inflammatory bowel disease, will contain bowel flora — especially Gram-negative organisms and anaerobes. Rarely, psoas abscesses arise from the genitourinary tract, suppurative iliac lymphadenitis or chest empyema.

4 In this case, all 3 sets of blood cultures yielded *Staphylococcus aureus* after 48 hours, sensitive to penicillin (MIC and MBC <0.1 mg/l) and cloxacillin (MIC and MBC 0.25 mg/l). Chest x-ray was normal and hepatitis B serology indicated past infection only. The original CT scan excluded intrahepatic abscess. Diagnostic percutaneous aspiration of the psoas yielded pus containing *S.aureus* only and initial smears and prolonged culture for *Mycobacterium tuberculosis* were negative, as was prolonged culture of several early morning specimens of urine and sputum.

5 Initial empirical management with intravenous cloxacillin 12 g/day was changed to benzyl penicillin 18 g/day when sensitivity tests become available. Penicillin is the drug of choice when *S. aureus* is sensitive. However, the patient continued to have daily spiking fever (**5**), which resolved only when the abscesses were definitively drained (**6**). Bilateral sump drains were inserted into the upper and lower poles of both abscesses under local anaesthetic and CT control (**7, 8**). Several litres of pus were drained over the next 5 days and intravenous antibiotics were maintained for a total of 4 weeks. On this regimen the patient's blood penicillin levels were 0.5 mg/l (trough) and 16 mg/l (1 hour post-dose) with bactericidal titres of 1:8 and >1:64, respectively.

The alternative procedure would have been laparotomy to drain the abscesses, and this is a good example of the role of interventional radiology in treating deep abscesses.

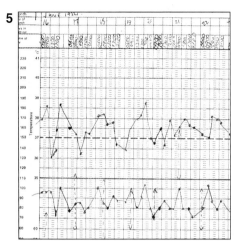

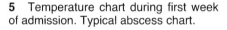

5 Temperature chart during first week of admission. Typical abscess chart.

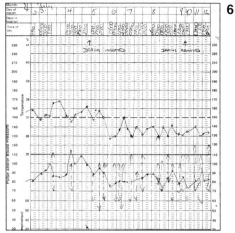

6 Resolution of fever after insertion of sump drains.

7 CT scan showing bilateral iliacus and psoas abscesses extending across the midline and displacing the aorta anteriorly.

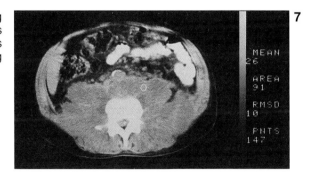

8 Post-drainage CT scan showing placement of one of the drains. Note marked decrease in size of the abscesses, and presence of gas in the abscess area from the drainage and irrigation.

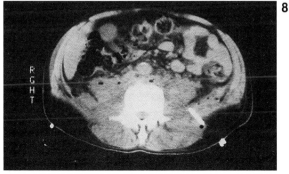

Case 5

Fever, rash and hypotension in an orthopaedic patient

History

A 59-year-old man is admitted for removal of the acromial process to relieve a persistent right frozen shoulder. Four days after the operation he complains of pain in the right shoulder and a sore throat. On examination his temperature is 39.5°C and he has marked pharyngeal inflammation. The operative wound is tender but not clinically infected. He is started on ampicillin 500 mg orally qid after blood and pharyngeal cultures are taken. The fever continues and 48 hours later he is found to be hypotensive and oliguric with a high fever. There is a slight exudate from the wound and a diffuse, blanching, generalised erythematous rash is present.

The ampicillin is discontinued, the wound is explored, and thin serosanguinous pus aspirated. Following the operation he is transferred to ITU. He has a temperature of 40.1°C , pulse of 156, systolic blood pressure of 75, and a respiratory rate of 35. In addition to the rash, he has generalised oedema (**1**), jaundice, and conjunctival injection (**2**).

Haematology:	Hb 12.5 g/dl WBC 20.5 × 10⁹/l Neutrophils 88%, lymphocytes 13%
Biochemistry:	Na 135 mmol/l K 5.2 mmol/l Urea 36.9 mmol/l Creatinine 809 µmol/l Bilirubin 63 µmol/l Alk. phos. 290 u/l ALT 205 u/l CK 1900 u/l
Microbiology:	Blood cultures: negative at 48 hours Throat culture: normal flora Gram stain of shoulder pus (**3**)
Chest x-ray:	Illustrated opposite (**4**)
Blood gases: *(60% oxygen)*	pO₂ 7.9 kPa (62 mmHg); pCO₂ 3.61 kPa (27 mmHg)

Questions

1 What does the Gram stain show?
2 What diagnosis would you consider to be most likely?
3 How would you confirm the diagnosis?
4 What treatment would you give?

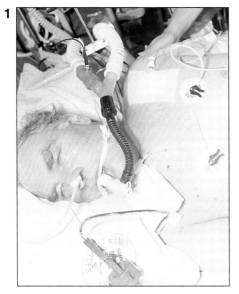

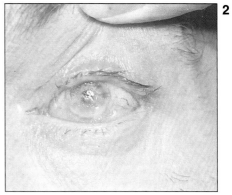

2 Conjunctival injection and jaundice.

1 Patient in ITU.

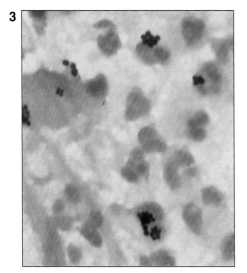

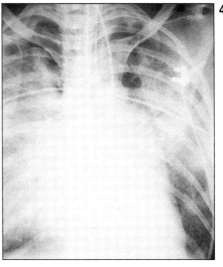

3 Gram stain of pus from shoulder.

4 Chest x-ray on admission to ITU.

Case 5

Answers

1   The Gram stain shows polymorphonuclear leucocytes and Gram-positive cocci in clusters. These are likely to be staphylococci.

2   The diagnosis initially entertained was fever and rash due to ampicillin allergy. As the patient's condition deteriorated in ITU, septicaemia with multiple organ dysfunction secondary to a staphylococcal wound infection seemed more probable. However, several features do not fit either diagnosis. In fact, this is staphylococcal toxic shock syndrome (Box 1). The onset is variable and fever for 4 days prior to onset of frank shock is not uncommon. Pharyngitis occurs in approximately two-thirds of cases and conjunctival injection is common. The erythematous rash is often subtle and relatively transient, and may first be noticed after the onset of shock. The laboratory findings of polymorphonuclear leucocytosis, deranged LFTs, elevated CK and renal failure are all compatible with severe toxic shock syndrome, as is the onset of adult respiratory distress syndrome suggested by the chest x-ray (4).

In the UK, about half of all cases of toxic shock are related to menstruation, while the remainder are associated with localised infections which can appear to be quite trivial. The majority of post-operative cases occur within 4 days of surgery but delays of greater than 1 month have been known. Approximately 10–15% of patients die.

3   Confirmation of the diagnosis depends on the isolation of *Staphylococcus aureus* from the vagina or other infected site and waiting for desquamation (10–21 days after onset). This is usually most marked on the hands and feet (5, 6).

Demonstration that the staphylococcal isolate produces one of the toxins associated with toxic shock syndrome in the laboratory is desirable but not essential. Most (90%) of menstrual cases are due to phage type I strains producing toxic shock syndrome toxin (TSST-1), while non-menstrual cases are often due to enterotoxin B producing strains of phage type V. Strains producing enterotoxins A or C are more rarely implicated and some isolates produce no detectable toxin.

4   Supportive care is usually provided on an ITU as ventilation and haemodialysis may be needed in severe cases. Eradication of infection, tampon removal or surgical exploration and drainage may be required in addition to antibiotics. Flucloxacillin is usually the agent of first choice with erythromycin as an alternative. Either should be given for at least 10 days. If carriage is not eliminated, a course of rifampicin with another antistaphylococcal agent can be tried as recurrent episodes are reported in menstrual toxic shock syndrome.

Neutralisation of toxin may be helpful in theory. Since most adults (75%) have antibodies to TSST-1, there is a rationale for giving pooled IV gamma globulin. However, there are currently no controlled data to support its use.

This patient survived with intensive inotrope support, ventilation and haemofiltration. He was discharged from the ITU after 14 days but required regular haemodialysis for a further month. Extensive desquamation of hands and feet occurred in convalescence (5, 6), but he eventually made a good recovery.

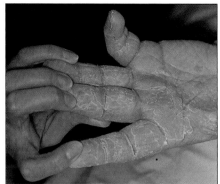

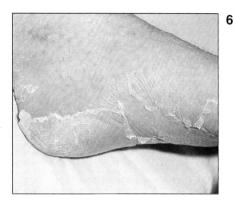

5, 6 Desquamation of hands and feet in convalescence.

Box 1: Toxic shock syndrome

Clinical case definition for Public Health surveillance (MMWR, 19 Oct 1990; **39** RR–13: 38–9)

An illness with the following clinical manifestations:

- Fever: temperature ≥ 38.9°C (102°F).
- Rash: diffuse macular erythroderma.
- Desquamation: 1–2 weeks after onset of illness, particularly palms and soles.
- Hypotension: systolic blood pressure ≤ 90 mmHg for adults (or less than fifth percentile by age for children <16 years of age), orthostatic drop in diastolic blood pressure ≥ 15 mmHg from lying to sitting, orthostatic syncope or orthostatic dizziness.
- Multisystem involvement: three or more of the following:
  gastrointestinal: vomiting or diarrhoea at onset of illness;
  muscular: severe myalgia or creatine phosphokinase level at least twice the upper limit of normal for laboratory;
  mucous membrane: vaginal, oropharyngeal or conjunctival hyperaemia;
  renal: blood urea nitrogen or creatinine at least twice the upper limit of normal for laboratory or urinary sediment with pyuria (≥5 leucocytes per high-power field) in the absence of urinary tract infection;
  hepatic: total bilirubin, serum AST or serum ALT at least twice the upper limit of normal for laboratory;
  haematological: platelets <100 × 10^9/l;
  central nervous system: disorientation or alterations in consciousness without focal neurological signs when fever and hypotension are absent.
- Negative results on the following tests, if obtained:
  blood, throat or cerebral fluid cultures (blood culture may be positive for Staphylococcus aureus);
  rise in titre to Rocky Mountain spotted fever, leptospirosis or measles.

Case classification

Probable: a case with five of the six clinical findings described above.
Confirmed: a case with all six of the clinical findings described above, including desquamation, unless the patient dies before desquamation could occur.

Case 6

Chronic back pain in an elderly woman

History

An 82-year-woman is admitted for investigation of back pain of 18 months duration. Initially, it was relieved by bed rest but recently this has made no difference and the pain now interferes with her sleep. As she is known to have osteoarthritis of the knee and hips, her back pain has been ascribed to this by her general practitioner and she has received a variety of non-steroidal anti-inflammatory agents over the last 2 years. Despite increasing doses they have ceased to relieve the pain. She has no medical history of note but her father died of pulmonary tuberculosis when she was 14 years old and one of her sisters spent 2 years in a tuberculosis sanatorium as a child.

On examination she is thin and has a back deformity (1). She is afebrile with a pulse of 84 and blood pressure of 175/95. There are no other abnormalities except for changes compatible with osteoarthritis in both knees.

Haematology:	Hb 11.7 g/dl WBC 8.7×10^9/l ESR 42 mm/hr
Biochemistry:	Na 135 mmol/l K 5.2 mmol/l Urea 23 mmol/l Creatinine 420 µmol/l
Radiology:	Ilustrated opposite (2–4)
Urine:	pH 8.0, blood +++, protein ++++ Microscopy: shown opposite (5, 6) Culture: illustrated on page 32 (7)

Questions

1 What abnormalities are shown on the x-rays?
2 What does the urine microscopy show?
3 What is the probable identity of the urinary pathogen and what simple test would confirm this?
4 What are the possible causes of the patient's renal failure?
5 What are the likely causes of her back problem?
6 What further tests would you suggest to confirm the diagnosis?

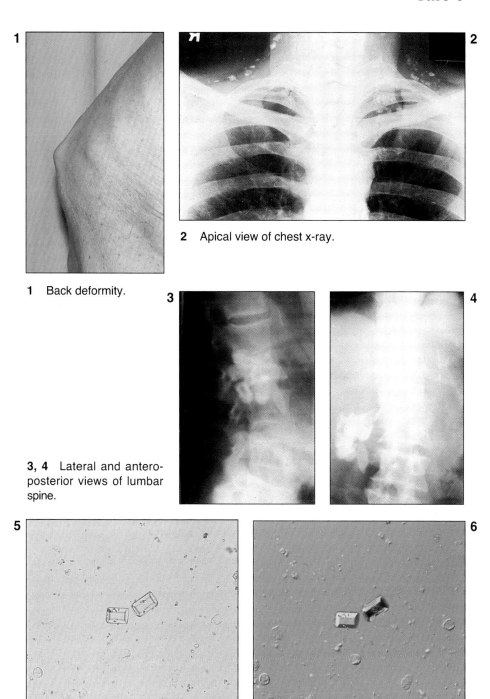

2 Apical view of chest x-ray.

1 Back deformity.

3, 4 Lateral and antero-posterior views of lumbar spine.

5, 6 Unstained microscopy (**5**) and Nomarski interference microscopy (**6**) of urine.

Case 6

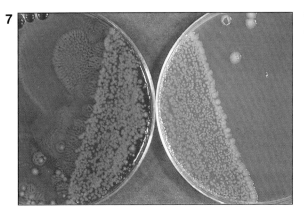

7 Aerobic cultures of urine on blood agar (left) and MacConkey's medium (right).

Answers

1   The apical chest view shows calcified glands in the neck and calcified foci in the apices, suggesting previous infection with tuberculosis. The lumbar spine x-rays reveal extensive calcification in the left kidney and the collapse of the second lumbar vertebra with erosion of the end plates of L1 and L3. The appearance suggests discitis and osteomyelitis.

2 and 3   The urine microscopy shows struvite (triple phosphate) crystals and numerous red cells, white cells and bacteria. The culture plates show discrete colonies of a non-lactose fermenting organism on MacConkey's medium and swarming of the organism on blood agar. These features are typical of *Proteus* sp. which split urea by production of urease, leading to a high urinary pH and subsequent struvite deposition. This can be confirmed by a urease test (**8**).

4   The renal calcification raises the possibility of renal tuberculosis, particularly in view of the patient's family history and the chest x-ray findings. Renal tuberculosis, alone, may account for renal failure if the disease is bilateral, especially if there are ureteric strictures and obstruction. Another possibility is that the calcification is a 'stag horn' type calculus secondary to struvite deposition, the result of chronic infection with a urea splitting organism. However, unilateral disease would not be expected to cause renal failure in the absence of another pathological process. The woman's drug history places her at risk of analgesic nephropathy and the likely chronicity of her renal infection raises the possibility of amyloidosis.

5   The back pain is probably due to vertebral osteomyelitis, although the renal disease may also be contributing. The most likely infecting organism is *Mycobacterium tuberculosis,* or a coliform (in this case, proteus) related to chronic urinary tract infection.

6   It is important to confirm that the *Proteus* sp. can be isolated repeatedly from mid-stream specimens of urine (MSSU). Proteus is often a contaminant, particularly in disabled or elderly patients who may not be able to co-operate well enough to provide a clean MSSU, in which case a catheter specimen should be obtained. Early morning urine specimens should also be collected on 3 successive days for mycobacterial stain and culture. Chronic urinary obstruction should be excluded by ultrasonography scan or IVU as this is potentially amenable to treatment.

Vertebral osteomyelitis caused by pyogenic organisms, most often

Case 6

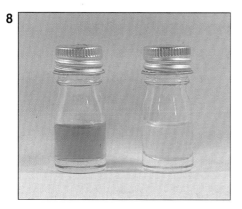

8 Urea broth inoculated with Proteus (left bottle). The purple colour indicates the presence of urease. Control broth on right.

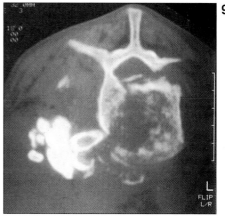

9 CT scan showing destruction of lumbar vertebral body and impingement of calcified renal stone.

Staphylococcus aureus or a coliform, is often a remarkably indolent process. The clinical features may be unimpressive and fever minimal; persistent back pain unrelieved by rest may be the only symptom. Pyogenic and tuberculous vertebral disease cannot be distinguished reliably on clinical grounds. Investigation usually reveals a raised ESR and imaging shows erosion of vertebral bodies on adjacent sides of a disc space. The only way to provide a definite diagnosis in this situation is to obtain material directly from the spine, either by closed aspiration under x-ray guidance or by open biopsy. Bacteraemic seeding of disc spaces is believed to be the first step in the pathogenesis of this disease and accounts for the higher rate of coliform infection in the elderly in whom urinary tract infection and degenerative disc disease are both relatively common. Direct erosion by a renal stone as in this case (**9**) is very uncommon.

Progress

Open biopsy of the spine confirmed extensive osteomyelitis and allowed sequestrum to be removed. Fragments of bone yielded a scanty growth of *Proteus* sp. sensitive to ampicillin and trimethoprim. Mycobacterial cultures were negative after 8 weeks incubation. Initially, high dose intravenous ampicillin was administered(2 g 6 hourly), followed by oral treatment for a total of 3 months to treat the bone infection. In view of the patient's frailty, the calcified kidney, which showed no function by nephrogram, was not removed but long-term suppressive antimicrobial therapy with trimethoprim 100 mg daily was instigated. In retrospect, it was noted that a *Proteus* sp. had been isolated from urine 2 years earlier. This had been treated but no follow-up urine cultures had been organised. If they had, the woman's later problems might have been avoided.

Case 7

Nosocomial pneumonia following renal transplantation

History

A 24-year-old man with a history of asthma and an episode of left lower lobe pneumonia 2 years earlier is admitted for cadaveric renal transplantation. The operation proceeds without complication and he maintains good renal function while receiving prednisolone and cyclosporin. However, on the 9th post-operative day he develops fever, headache, diarrhoea and malaise. On examination his temperature is 39.4°C but he has no signs suggestive of focal infection. Blood cultures are taken but no sputum is available for culture and he is started on amoxycillin. The fever continues and on chest auscultation 48 hours later he is found to have crackles in the right mid-zone and axilla. A chest radiograph is taken (**1**).

Treatment is changed to cefotaxime 1 g tid. After a further 72 hours there is no improvement and a repeat radiograph is taken (**2**).

Haematology:	Hb 11.4 g/dl
	WBC 11.8 × 10⁹/l
	Neutrophils 80%, lymphocytes 17%
Biochemistry:	Na 145 mmol/l
	K 5.2 mmol/l
	Urea 22 mmol/l
	Creatinine 238 μmol/l
Microbiology:	Blood culture: no growth at 5 days
	Sputum on 14th post-operative day: microscopy (**3**) and culture (**4, 5**)

Questions

1 What additional investigations would you ask for and how would you interpret the sputum microbiology results?
2 What changes would you make to the antimicrobial treatment at this stage?
3 Are there any infection control measures to be taken at this stage?

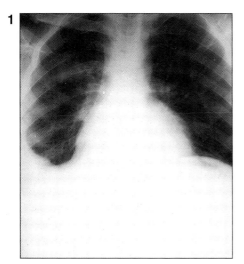
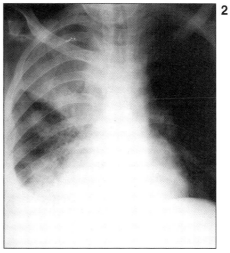

1 Chest x-ray, 11th post-operative day. **2** Chest x-ray 72 hours later.

3 Gram stain of sputum (high power).

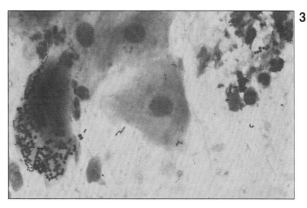

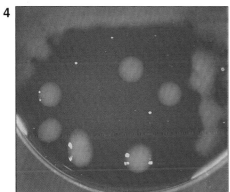
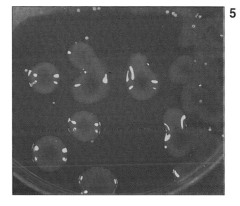

4, 5 Sputum culture after 48 hours on blood agar (**4**) and MacConkey's medium (**5**).

Case 7

Answers

1 The onset of pneumonia 9 days after an operation when the patient is ambulant and can cough without pain suggests that this is not simply related to aspiration and impaired mucus clearance, the predisposing factors for post-operative pneumonia. The lack of response to cefotaxime and progressive lobar infiltration are also unusual in post-operative pneumonia due to typical pathogens.

The sputum microscopy shows several buccal epithelial cells and Gram-negative rods which are not associated with polymorphs. The culture reveals an absence of normal buccal flora, but the presence of small colonies of yeasts and a heavy growth of a mucoid lactose-fermenting coliform, which was later identified as *Klebsiella pneumoniae*. The recovery of coliforms from the sputum of hospitalised patients (especially while on antibiotics) and from poor samples with a high salivary content is very common and rarely reflects the infective process in the lung. Even when a possible pathogen such as *K. pneumoniae* is recovered, this should not be regarded as the definite cause of the infection. Infection by opportunists such as *Pneumocystis carinii* or CMV is unlikely so soon after transplantation.

Among the atypical pathogens, *Legionella pneumophila* is the most likely in the context of a nosocomial pneumonia in an adult, particularly one receiving immunosuppressive therapy. Legionellosis is diagnosed most often by serology, which is sometimes positive as early as day 4 of the infection. A positive serological result from an acute serum sample is helpful but a diagnostic rise in titre often takes several weeks to develop. An alternative approach in early infection is to test urine for the presence of legionella antigen. While *Legionella* sp. grow slowly (72 hours) and require special media, such as buffered charcoal yeast extract (BCYE) (**6**), their isolation and subsequent serogrouping can be useful in investigating the source of the infection. Sputum culture for legionella would be worthwhile but the yield would be better from bronchial lavage which should be strongly considered. Very rarely, *Legionella* sp. can be recovered from blood culture. This may be missed since little CO_2 is generated and systems relying on this will not identify growth. Routine subculture will detect growth only if the correct media are employed.

2 Intravenous erythromycin should be added to cover atypical pathogens and the cefotaxime could be discontinued as there has clearly been progression in the pneumonia during its administration.

3 No infection control measures are necessary at this stage beyond checking that there has been no increased frequency of pneumonia either on the patient's ward or among recently discharged patients. If it has been confirmed that the patient had legionellosis, it would be essential to investigate the possible sources of the infection. For the majority of the incubation period (2–14 days) he was in hospital, so it is necessary to record where he has been – which rooms, baths, showers, theatres, etc. The source of legionella is mainly water aerosols, so wet air-conditioning units (**7**) and showers need the closest scrutiny. Taps, ice makers, and drinking water are less likely sources, but in the rooms where the patient was resident it would nevertheless be advisable to check them all (**8**). There is no recognised risk of person-to-person transmission of *Legionella* sp.

The patient was found to have a reciprocal titre of 128 to legionella by indirect immunofluoresence. The titre in serum saved on admission in the blood bank was <16, confirming current legionnaires disease. His blood cultures were subcultured onto BCYE agar after 10 days and *L. pneumophila* serogroup 6 was recovered. A similar isolate was recovered from the shower which he had used on the day of admission. The patient made an uneventful recovery on erythromycin 1 g qid for 21 days.

6 Legionella growth on BCYE.

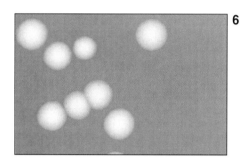
6

7 Wet air-conditioning unit – a typical reservoir of infection.

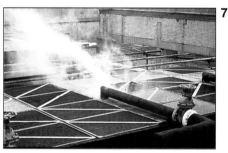
7

8 Culture of mixed Legionella sp. on BCYE viewed under UV light. Some non-pathogenic species autofluoresce but L. pneumophila does not. A rapid test to eliminate non-pathogenic Legionella sp. in environmental samples.

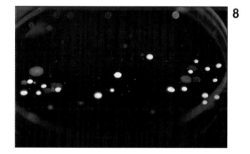
8

Case 8

Pyrexia of unknown origin

History

A 36-year-old woman of Lebanese descent is referred with a 3-month history of fever, malaise, arthralgia and pleuritic chest pains. She reports that the fever is usually worse in the evenings and on several occasions during the first month of the illness she has noticed a mildly pruritic patchy rash over the trunk and arms that invariably clears by the morning. She has lost 8 kg in weight.

On examination she is thin and has slight swelling of the right knee and elbow. These joints have full mobility despite some pain on movement. Her temperature is 39.5°C, pulse 105 and blood pressure 130/85. There is 1–2 cm mobile, non-tender lymphadenopathy in both axillae and the neck, but there are no other abnormal findings. One evening, two weeks after admission her rash reappears (1). Her temperature chart for the preceding week is shown in Figure 2. On careful review of her notes you find that, despite extensive investigation, no definite diagnosis has been reached. The only abnormalities discovered so far are:

Haematology:	Hb 8.9 g/dl, Hct 0.266, reticulocytes 5%
	WBC 38.1× 10^9/l
	Neutrophils 87% with left shift
	Platelets 754 × 10^9/l
	ESR 74 mm/hr
Biochemistry:	Alk. phos. 135 u/l/
	AST 256 u/l/
	γGT 154 u/l
	Albumin 28 g/l, total protein 73 g/l
Immunology:	Polyclonal increase in IgG and IgM
	C-reactive protein 234 mg/l
Lymph node biopsy:	Reactive changes

Questions

1 What further points in her history would you particularly ask about?
2 What investigations would you check had already been performed to investigate her pyrexia?
3 What diagnosis does the history, rash and fever chart suggest?
4 What additional investigations might be performed to confirm this clinical diagnosis?
5 What treatment would you consider starting?
6 What condition(s) would you be eager to exclude prior to starting this treatment?

1 Rash on arm of patient.

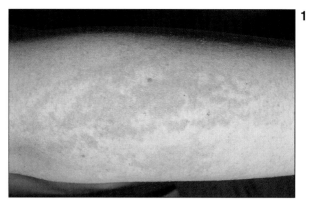

1

2 Temperature chart during second week of admission.

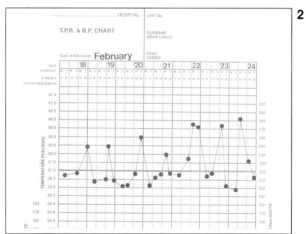

2

Answers

1 This woman's illness falls within the classic definition of 'pyrexia of unknown origin' (PUO) - a fever whose origin remains unknown after a week's investigation in hospital and which persists for 3 weeks with a temperature regularly exceeding 38.2°C. The leading causes of PUO are listed in Box 1.

A detailed history is critical in reaching a diagnosis and points which demand careful enquiry include:

- Travel history to assess whether she may be at risk of uncommon chronic infections, such as brucellosis, trypanosomiasis or leishmaniasis, which have defined high-risk zones.
- Family history, especially in view of her origin - which should suggest the possibility of familial Mediterranean fever.
- Drug history. Drug-related fever must always be considered, particularly in the presence of a rash. A trial of complete withdrawal of medication may be necessary.
- HIV risk behaviour history. The approach to PUO is radically altered in a patient with HIV-related immunodeficiency.

Case 8

Box 1: causes of classical PUO

(Petersdorf RG and Beeson PG.
N. Engl. J. Med.,1961; **40**: 1–30)

Infections:	Cryptic abscesses (NB pelvic and dental)
	Osteomyelitis
	Endocarditis
	Tuberculosis
	Yersiniosis
	Epstein–Barr virus
	Cytomegalovirus infection
	Toxoplasmosis
Neoplasms:	Lymphomas, leukaemias
	Hypernephroma
	Hepatoma
	Atrial myxoma
	Phaeochromo-cytoma

Collagen, vascular diseases:	Systemic lupus erythematosus (SLE)
	Polyarteritis nodosa
	Giant cell arteritis
	Rheumatoid arthritis
	Polymyalgia rheumatica
	Other types of vasculitis
Granulomatous diseases:	Granulomatous hepatitis
	Sarcoidosis
	Crohn's disease
Miscellaneous:	Drug fever
	Familial Mediter-ranean fever
	Hypothalamic disorders
	Factitious fever
	Pulmonary embolism

Box 2: investigations in PUO

Those marked * would be suggested by clinical findings and should not be part of an initial screen.

Full blood count and differential
ESR and C-reactive protein
Tests of kidney, liver and thyroid function
Urine microscopy and culture (including AFB if pyuria present)
Blood cultures: three sets on separate occasions
Sputum, if available, for mycobacterial culture
Tuberculin testing
Immunoglobulins and complement
Autoantibody screen, in particular antinuclear antibodies, DNA binding and rheumatoid factor
Anti-neutrophil cytoplasmic antibodies
*Serum angiotensin-converting enzyme
*Serology for brucellosis, yersiniosis, chlamydia, coxiella, syphilis, hepatitis B and C, and HIV
Imaging; chest x-ray, IVU, abdominal ultrasound, *abdominal CTor MR scan
*Isotope scanning; bone scan, Gallium scan, Indium labelled WBC scan
*Biopsies; bone marrow, lymph node, liver

2   The diagnostic work-up of a patient with PUO must be guided by clinical clues but would usually include the investigations listed in Box 2.

3   The combination of an evanescent rash and high fever in the evening with a return to normal by morning is typical of adult Still's disease. The main features of this condition are given in Box 3. The particular importance of Still's disease in infectious disease practice is that the leucocytosis and fever invariably raise the possibility of cryptic infection and set in train an extensive series of negative investigations. Abnormal liver

---

Box 3: features of adult Still's disease

Case definition:*
High spiking fever >39°C often peaks in evening
Arthralgia or arthritis
Negative rheumatoid factor <1:80
Negative antinuclear factor <1:100

And any two of:

Leucocytosis >15 × 10⁹/l, usually with neutrophilia
Evanescent macular or maculopapular rash
Serositis: pleuritis or pericarditis
Recticuloendothelial involvement: hepatomegaly, splenomegaly, lymphadenopathy

Other clinical features include: myalgia, sore throat, weight loss, pneumonitis, abdominal pain.

Other laboratory features include: anaemia Hb <10 g/l, ESR >30 mm/hr, albumin <35 g/l, elevated liver enzymes.

*After Medsger and Christy in Cush, JJ et al., Arthritis and Rheumatism, 1987; **30**: 186–194.

---

enzymes are also a common feature. Liver biopsy usually shows non-specific reactive changes only.

4   There are no diagnostic tests which confirm a clinical diagnosis of Still's disease, although a raised serum ferritin level is supportive. This patient had a serum ferritin of 8704 ng/ml (normal range 10–300). As diagnostic tests have improved, the spectrum of causes of PUO has shifted; following the introduction of tests for anti-nuclear factor and DNA-binding antibodies, SLE is usually diagnosed early in the course of investigations. The improvement in intra-abdominal images obtained by ultrasound, CT scanning or magnetic resonance imaging has resulted in the earlier diagnosis of cryptic abscesses and malignancies. As a consequence, Still's disease has become a more frequent (but still relatively rare) cause of classical PUO.

5   While Still's disease may respond to high doses of aspirin or other non-steroidal anti-inflammatory drugs, steroids are often required to induce remission which may take several weeks. This patient responded to steroids after 2 weeks.

6   Prior to commencing steroids it is particularly important to consider tuberculosis. Cryptic TB is difficult to exclude, and in a patient with less convincing clinical features of Still's it may be advisable to perform a liver biopsy before commencing a trial of steroids. While blind liver biopsy will not totally exclude TB, it has a higher sensitivity than any other investigation – including bone-marrow biopsy for disseminated TB. It is essential to culture the biopsy, as Ziehl–Neelsen tissue stains may be negative despite positive subsequent culture. Non-specific granulomatous changes on liver biopsy also have a wide differential diagnosis. The chest x-ray should be repeated after 2 to 3 weeks since miliary shadowing of TB sometimes becomes apparent later in the illness. If in doubt, steroid treatment of the patient may need to be 'covered' with specific antituberculous therapy.

Case 9

Floaters

Case A

A 30-year-old man (1) travelled to Leningrad (now St Petersburg) for a short holiday. Two weeks after his return he developed diarrhoea which continued despite antispasmodics prescribed by his general practitioner. One sample of faeces sent to another laboratory was reported as showing 'no enteropathogens on culture' and 'negative faecal microscopy'. After 2 more weeks he attends clinic with symptoms of vague malaise, abdominal bloating and nausea. As soon as he gets out of bed in the morning he rushes to the toilet and 'explodes'. He opens his bowels several more times in the morning, describing the motions as flecks of porridge-like material with an offensive smell, sticking to the toilet pan. He has lost 5 kg in weight.

Case B

A 21-year-old man is admitted for intravenous antibiotic treatment of a lung abscess caused by *Streptococcus milleri* (2). He has been subject to recurrent chest infections, due mainly to *Haemophilus influenzae*, since early childhood and has a chronic cough productive of up to a cupful of sputum per day. Following investigations at the age of 10, he has been receiving intramuscular and, more recently, intravenous treatment on a monthly basis and family members have been taught to administer chest physiotherapy with postural drainage twice a day.

Following successful treatment of his lung abscess he is referred to a gastroenterologist for investigation of intermittent offensive pale diarrhoea from which he has been suffering for several months, predating his lung abscess treatment. Characteristic appearances are seen on endoscopy of the upper intestine (3). Figure 4 shows a low-power view of a duodenal biopsy taken at endoscopy.

Questions

1 What organisms are likely to be causing these two patients' diarrhoea?
2 Why is the travel history of the first patient relevant?
3 What are the possible underlying reasons for the chronic chest problem of the second patient?
4 What does the endoscopy show?
5 What procedure is being carried out on patient A? (1)
6 What other investigations are likely to be appropriate?
7 How would you treat these patients?

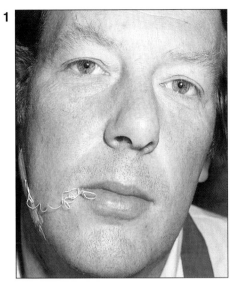

1 The traveller (Case A).

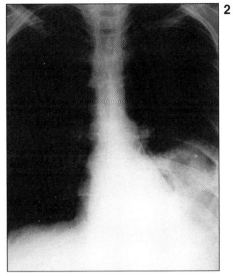

2 Chest x-ray of second patient.

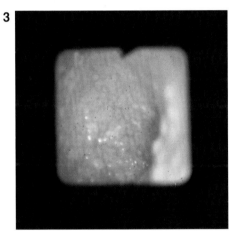

3 Endoscopic view of duodenum of second patient.

4 Low-power view of duodenal biopsy.

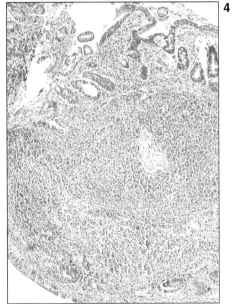

Case 9

Answers

1 and 2   Both patients have diarrhoea persisting for over a month and one has a history of travel to a city notorious for endemicity of *Giardia lamblia* and cryptosporidiosis due to contamination of its water supply by sewage. Giardiasis is the commonest infectious cause of chronic diarrhoea in travellers to the tropics and other endemic areas, and the symptoms described by the first patient are typical. The infection is also commonly found in children and adults without a history of exotic travel, particularly if the child attends day-care facilities. Other parasites to consider include *Isospora belli, Cryptosporidium* sp. and *Cyclospora* sp., all of which cause more severe illness in HIV-positive patients in whom microsporidial infection should also be excluded. The differential diagnosis includes other causes of malabsorption, especially tropical sprue, coeliac disease and alcohol abuse.

3 and 4   The second patient has bronchiectasis. This could be due to cystic fibrosis or secondary to common acquired hypogammaglobulinaemia (Bruton's disease). The latter usually predisposes to *H. influenzae* infections, which also complicate cystic fibrosis, but a cystic fibrosis patient is likely to have become colonised by *Pseudomonas* sp. by the age of 20. Specific questioning revealed that his brother also had Bruton's disease and that he has recently been receiving intravenous immunoglobulin. His endoscopy reveals nodular lymphoid hyperplasia, which is sometimes a normal variant but is more common in patients with hypogammaglobulinaemia and the subgroup with coeliac disease combined with IgA deficiency. Trophozoites of *G. lamblia* can be seen at higher magnification(**5**). Patients with Bruton's disease often harbour *G. lamblia,* which intermittently causes diarrhoea, and this phenomenon has recently been reported in those with cystic fibrosis. Since this patient has received multiple courses of antibiotics, *Clostridium difficile* associated diarrhoea should also be excluded by faecal culture of faeces and their examination for toxin.

5 and 6   There are several reasons for failing to diagnose *G. lamblia* infection. The usual method is examination of a wet preparation of faeces for cysts or trophozoites, and concentration of faeces for specific staining such as trichrome or iodine (**6, 7**). However, cyst excretion is irregular and multiple successive faecal samples can be negative. Trophozoites are usually seen only in the faeces of patients with brisk diarrhoea and are sometimes mistaken for *Trichomonas* sp. by less experienced observers. If the laboratory is not given full clinical details, faecal examination is likely to be inadequate. It is particularly important to exclude giardiasis in patients with malabsorption, especially in the case of children being investigated for possible coeliac disease.

If adequate faecal examination remains negative, specific diagnostic options include jejunal/duodenal biopsy by Crosby capsule or at upper gastrointestinal endoscopy, or a string test which is less invasive and can be performed in the clinic. The first patient has swallowed an Enterotest® capsule after an overnight fast (**8**). This dissolves in the stomach and the weighted end of the string is carried through the duodenum within a couple of hours, at which point the patient usually feels peristaltic tugging on the end of the string. Our practice is to leave the string *in situ* for a further 90

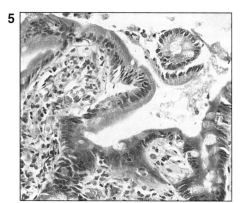

5 High-power view of duodenal biopsy, showing trophozoites of Giardia lamblia and flattening of villi (haematoxylin & eosin).

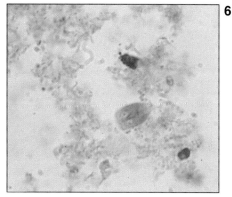

6 Trichrome stain of faeces, showing trophozoites (size 6–10 μm × 10–20 μm).

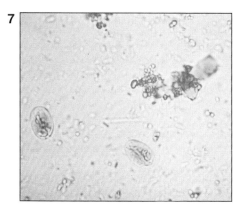

7 Typical appearance of G. lamblia cysts in iodine-stained wet preparation of faeces (size 5 × 10–14 μm).

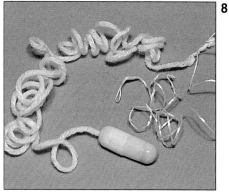

8 Enterotest® capsule (string test).

minutes and then pull it out (**9**). The bile-stained juice can be stripped off the string (1–2 ml yield) (**10**) or the bile-stained portion of the string may be cut off into 1–3 ml of normal saline to be sent to the laboratory. Immediate examination reveals active trophozoites of *G. lamblia*, which can be stained after drying the slide. In our experience, this technique is more sensitive than examination of duodenal aspirate fluid. Serological tests, faecal antigen assays and specific antibody-based stains for *G. lamblia* have not yet become accepted for individual patient diagnosis.

Case 9

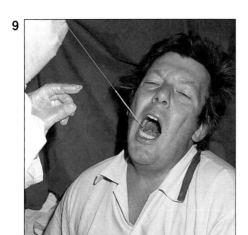

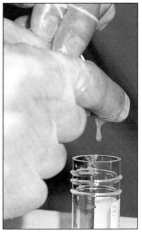

9, 10 Removal of string by steady pull takes 1–2 seconds. The discomfort is short-lived! The bile-stained portion of the string yields 1–2 ml of fluid.

Supportive investigations include features of malabsorption in the full blood count (anaemia, high MCV due to folate or vitamin B_{12} deficiency), serum biochemistry (low albumin) and small bowel meal (non-specific flocculation), but these features are usually absent in milder cases. Patients with recurrent or refractory giardiasis should be questioned carefully about travel and contact history, family history and other risk factors for immunosuppression, including sexual practices. Specific investigations should include measurement of serum immunoglobulin levels and HIV testing may be appropriate, although *G. lamblia* is not usually a more severe infection in HIV-positive individuals than in seronegative patients.

7   Treatment can be effected with metronidazole 2 g on 3 successive days or a single 2 g dose of tinidazole, or by 5 days of metronidazole 400 mg tid. Mepacrine is not used as first-line treatment in the UK but is still recommended in the USA. Although albendazole has been reported to be effective, its use for giardiasis has not yet found wide acceptance. The success of therapy can be gauged by symptomatic response alone in most patients. Although imidazole resistance has been reported for *G. lamblia*, this is rarely the reason for apparent therapeutic failure, which is often due to non-compliance and the patient should be questioned about this before starting a second course. Temporary intestinal lactase deficiency commonly occurs, and patients requiring a second course of treatment should be advised to avoid any milky products (including lactose-based medications) for 2 weeks. If these measures do not succeed it is likely that reinfection is occurring from other family members who may not be symptomatic (especially children) and treatment of the whole family may therefore be necessary. Outbreaks of *G. lamblia* in day-care facilities require full investigation and remedial measures. The parasite cysts are relatively resistant to chlorination, so additional filtering and chlorination of the water supply may be necessary.

Case 10

A diabetic with abdominal pain

History

A 25-year-old woman with a 10-year history of insulin-dependent diabetes mellitus is admitted to hospital with a 3-day history of fever, chills and left-sided flank pain. She has a history of recurrent urinary tract infections but no other recognised diabetic complications. She had consulted her general practitioner 2 days earlier and been given oral amoxycillin 250 mg 8 hourly for suspected urinary tract infection. On examination she has a temperature of 39.5°C, pulse of 110, and her blood pressure is 105/60. She has marked tenderness in the right flank and renal angle. An IVU is performed (1).

Haematology:	Hb 12.2 g/dl WBC 19.7×10^9/l Neutrophils 88% with left shift
Biochemistry:	Na 139 mmol/l, K 5.2 mmol/l Urea 16 mmol/l, Creatinine 130 µmol/l Glucose 22.5 mmol/l
Blood gases: *(room air)*	pH 7.2, pO_2 13.5 kPa (101 mmHg), pCO_2 3.8 kPa (29 mmHg) standard HCO_3 9 mmol/l, base excess -16 mmol/l

Questions

1 What abnormality is shown on the IVU film (1)?
2 What does the urine microscopy show (2)?
3 What is the most likely diagnosis?
4 What additional investigations would you perform?
5 What treatment would you initiate?

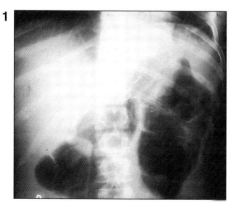

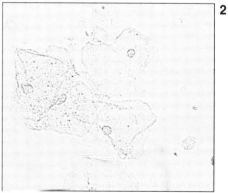

1 Intravenous urogram. View taken 10 minutes after contrast injection.

2 Microscopy of mid-stream urine specimen.

Case 10

Answers

1   There is gas in the tissues surrounding the left kidney which is not excreting contrast. This is seen more clearly on the CT scan (3).

2   The urine contains numerous epithelial cells. This suggests a poorly collected sample which is likely to yield a growth of vulvo-vaginal flora. The absence of numerous neutrophils is unusual in symptomatic urinary tract infection but may occur if there is obstruction of the outflow of urine from an infected kidney or if the infection is purely perinephric. When a reliable result is urgently required from a seriously ill patient who cannot provide a clean MSSU, it is essential to collect a sample by passing a urinary catheter or by suprapubic aspiration. The catheter should be left in only if it is required for other reasons.

3   The diagnosis is emphysematous pyelonephritis. This is an uncommon but serious complication of coliform urinary tract infection, found almost exclusively in patients with diabetes mellitus. Cultures usually yield a pure growth of *Escherichia coli* which cannot be distinguished from isolates causing uncomplicated pyelonephritis. Gas formation appears to be related to high blood/urinary sugar, possibly complicated by papillary necrosis and obstruction. *E. coli* characteristically produces gas *in vitro* (4).

4   Blood must be taken for culture before starting further antibiotics. Surgical intervention is usually required in this condition and nephrectomy and debridement of surrounding tissues is often the only option. Additional imaging such as CT scanning may be helpful in pre-operative assessment.

5   Her diabetes must be controlled as rapidly as possible with appropriate intravenous fluids and insulin. Antimicrobial chemotherapy should be started to give comprehensive cover of coliforms. Amoxycillin or trimethoprim are inadequate in such a serious infection as the risk of encountering a resistant isolate is too high, even in community-acquired infection. Resistance to cefuroxime is also sufficiently common to make this agent unsuitable in this situation. A third-generation cephalosporin, co-amoxyclav, a fluoroquinolone, a carbapenem or an aminoglycoside, would be better choices. Early referral for surgical evaluation is essential.

Progress

She was given cefotaxime and a percutaneous drain was inserted into the gaseous cavity (5), and she subsequently underwent nephrectomy. This problem might have been avoided by better control of her diabetes and more active management of previous urinary tract infections, including prophylaxis with low-dose nitrofurantoin or trimethoprim.

3 CT scan of abdomen, showing distorted and displaced left renal shadow surrounded by gas which extends to right side.

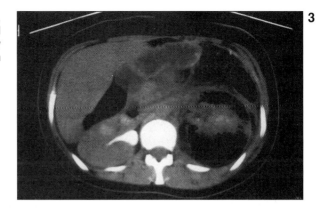

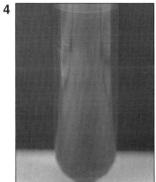

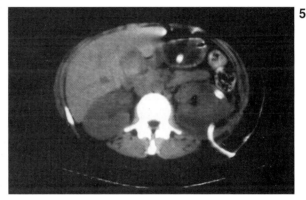

4 Durham's tube showing gas formation by Escherichia coli in glucose broth.

5 CT scan performed after percutaneous drainage of perinephric gas.

Case 11

The canary and the jailbird

History

A 23-year-old female nightclub singer is referred to the clinic with a 1-week history of malaise, vague fever, epigastric discomfort, nausea and pale diarrhoea. Two days prior to clinic attendance she developed pain in her right knee and the small joints of her left hand, and her boyfriend had noticed that her eyes looked yellow. She had not felt like smoking her usual 15 cigarettes a day. She denies any illicit drug use but admits to drinking several pints of cider on most evenings. She had a legal termination of pregnancy 3 weeks ago and has been taking a new oral contraceptive pill since then.

On examination she looks lethargic and has obvious jaundice with a rash on her trunk (**1**). Her temperature is slightly raised at 37.6°C. Her liver is palpable 2 cm below the costal margin but she has no detectable splenomegaly. There is no swelling of her joints, although passive movement of her right knee causes mild discomfort. Her muscles are not tender and there are no features of encephalopathy. Her urine specimen is shown opposite (**2**). Admission blood tests show:

Haematology: Hb 11.5 g/dl
WBC 6×10^9/l
Neutrophils 55%, lymphocytes 48%, monocytes 7%, eosinophils 5%
Platelets 148×10^9/l

Biochemistry: Bilirubin 248 μmol/l
AST 636 u/l
γGT 500 u/l
Alk. phos. 242 u/l
Prothrombin ratio (INR) 1.2
Albumin 38 g/l, total protein 70 g/l

Further questioning reveals that she has lived with her 30-year-old boyfriend, together with her 3-year-old son and 18-month-old daughter from a previous relationship, for 4 months. The children are cared for during the day by the singer's mother, who also 'baby sits' other small children in the same house. Her boyfriend has never had jaundice or a hepatitis-like illness but admits to heavy abuse of intravenous drugs in the past. He is not jaundiced but has the physical signs shown opposite (**3**, **4**). A sample of his blood shows:

Biochemistry: Bilirubin 35 μmol/l
AST 187 u/l
Alk. phos. 170 u/l
Albumin 40 g/l, total protein 72 g/l
Prothrombin ratio (INR) 1.1

Questions

1 What are the possible causes of the singer's illness?
2 What further questions should be asked of both singer and boyfriend?
3 What serological tests are indicated?
4 If your suspicions are correct, what management will be appropriate for her and her boyfriend?
5 What are the implications for the grandmother and the children?

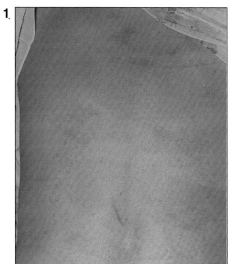

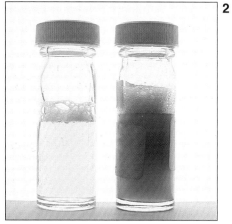

2 Urine of patient (right) compared to normal.

1 Faint confluent macular rash on back of jaundiced singer.

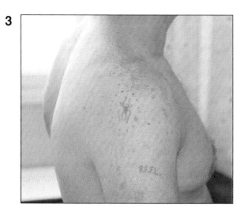

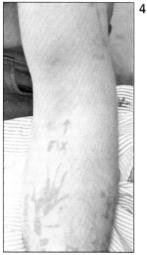

3 Right shoulder of boyfriend.

4 Left arm of boyfriend.

Case 11

Answers

1 and 2   The singer's symptoms are typical of acute hepatitis, with several possible aetiologies. The most likely diagnosis is that she has acquired hepatitis B from her boyfriend, who is a chronic hepatitis B carrier, suggested by the presence of spider naevi and his abnormal liver function tests. The usual incubation period for acute hepatitis B is 3–6 months. Transient rashes and joint pains occur in all forms of viral hepatitis, but are more common in the early stage of hepatitis B, presumably due to immune complex disease. Chronic carriage of hepatitis B follows 5–10% of acute infections and is more likely if the initial infection is asymptomatic.

Both patients were questioned further about other sexual contacts, whether these were protected by condom use, and whether any other sexual contacts were known to have, or be at risk of acquiring, hepatitis B. The boyfriend denied any homosexual contacts or sharing needles and there was no known liver disease or hepatitis in his own family. Neither patient had received a blood transfusion, had a tattoo, acupuncture or dental treatment in the preceding 9 months.

The presence of young children in the same house raised the possibility of hepatitis A, which in childhood is often very mild or asymptomatic and declares its presence when a non-immune adult member of the family develops overt hepatitis. Positive hepatitis C serology is common in IV drug abusers and the singer could have acquired this sexually from her boyfriend. However, the long-term risk of infection with a regular sexual partner is currently thought to be less than 5%, although still higher than the general population. Hepatitis E is unlikely in the absence of travel to the tropics.

Other infectious causes of hepatitis include Epstein–Barr virus, CMV, toxoplasmosis, leptospirosis and syphilis. She admits to drinking dangerous amounts of alcohol, and alcoholic hepatitis should be high in the differential diagnosis. Although the liver function tests are more hepatitic than cholestatic, liver damage caused by her recent anaesthetic or the contraceptive pill should be considered, and use of ecstasy (MDMA) should also be excluded. Surgical causes of jaundice such as cholelithiasis should not be forgotten.

3   Serological tests shown in Box 1 confirmed that both were hepatitis B positive, the singer with acute hepatitis B and the boyfriend with presumed chronic hepatitis B, suggested by the lack of anti-HBc IgM (although this may be present in up to 15% of chronic carriers). Recent hepatitis A was excluded but the boyfriend has had previous infections with hepatitis A and C (5). Tests for hepatitis C are unsatisfactory but PCR tests for viral RNA should assist in defining whether patients are still infected. Neither had been exposed to hepatitis D. Both patients were notified to the local CCDC.

4   The singer was admitted for 5 days' observation until her nausea had settled. Ultrasonography excluded obstructive biliary disease. The rash disappeared within 2 days but she developed severe pruritus, which responded to cholestyramine. No specific treatment has been shown to reduce the duration or histological severity of acute hepatitis or HBsAg excretion, and management is symptomatic. The most important aspect of management is to detect the small proportion of patients (about 2% of those

Box 1: serological tests

	Singer	Boyfriend
anti-HAV IgM	−	−
anti-HAV IgG	−	+
HBsAg	+	+
anti-HBs	−	−
anti-HBc IgM	+	−
anti-HBc IgG	−	+
HBeAg	+	+
anti-HBe	−	−
anti-HCV	−	+
anti-HDV	−	−

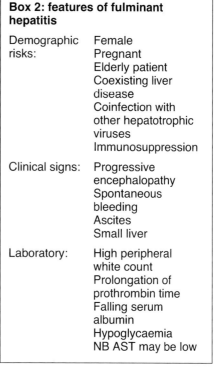

Box 2: features of fulminant hepatitis

Demographic risks:	Female Pregnant Elderly patient Coexisting liver disease Coinfection with other hepatotrophic viruses Immunosuppression
Clinical signs:	Progressive encephalopathy Spontaneous bleeding Ascites Small liver
Laboratory:	High peripheral white count Prolongation of prothrombin time Falling serum albumin Hypoglycaemia NB AST may be low

5

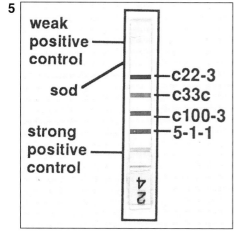

5 Second-generation RIBA (Ortho) strip from boyfriend, positive for hepatitis C. All four antigen bands (labelled on right) are darker than the control bands at either end (labelled on left). The band labelled 'sod' (superoxide dismutase) should not react, which is why it is not visible. (The yellow discolouration at the end is due to adhesive-tape.)

admitted to hospital) who develop fulminant hepatitis and who require intensive treatment – which may include emergency liver transplantation (Box 2).

The boyfriend had a normal serum alphafetoprotein and negative HIV tests. Ultrasonography of his liver showed a non-specific echobright pattern and endoscopy did not reveal oesophageal varices. Liver biopsy confirmed chronic active hepatitis B (6, 7). He was considered to be a good candidate for α-interferon treatment, with a roughly 40% chance of losing HBeAg, permanently reducing circulating HBV-DNA levels, and reducing the risk of further progression of liver disease (Box 3, overleaf). He received 10 Mu (6 Mu/m²) of recombinant α-interferon subcutaneously 3 times a week for 3 months but failed to develop an acute seroconversion illness or lose HBeAg positivity. He declined to prolong the interferon treatment because of side

Case 11

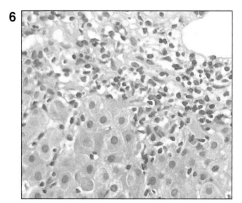
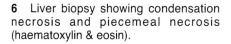

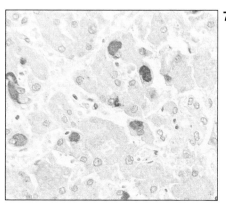

6 Liver biopsy showing condensation necrosis and piecemeal necrosis (haematoxylin & eosin).

7 Immunohistological stain, showing intracellular HBsAg as dark brown areas in hepatocytes.

effects of lethargy and difficulty concentrating. The optimal dose, duration and preparation of α-interferon for chronic active hepatitis B is still not fully established, but the above regimen is near the upper range of those shown to be effective.

5 Both the grandmother and the two children are in close contact with a known HBeAg-positive carrier and should be offered active prophylaxis with an accelerated course of hepatitis B vaccination (0, 1 month, 2 months and 12 months). Their risk of acquiring hepatitis B from the boyfriend is less than 5%, but would be higher if he was leaving used needles around the house. There is more risk to the children from the newly infected mother, although she was not breast-feeding her toddler. Specific hepatitis B immunoglobulin (HBIG) may also be given to high-risk contacts if seen within a week of onset of jaundice in the index case, but this advice applies mainly to sexual and needle contacts, and would not be appropriate in this case. In theory, the children could have serological tests for prior immunity to hepatitis B, but this is probably unnecessary. The other children cared for by the grandmother do not require vaccination.

Outcome

The singer was advised to remain off the contraceptive pill until her transaminases returned to normal. Serum HBeAg assay became negative at 2 months and by 4 months she was anti-HBe antibody positive and HBsAg negative. Prospective studies have failed to show a deleterious effect of moderate alcohol consumption on the outcome of uncomplicated acute viral hepatitis, but she was advised not to take any alcohol for 6 months because of her previous excessive intake. She and her boyfriend were advised on blood/secretion precautions, including instructions not to share toothbrushes with the other members of the family. The boyfriend remains under follow-up 3 years later with unchanged biochemistry or serology. He did not heed advice to use condoms with other partners and a casual sexual contact of his developed acute hepatitis B 1 year later.

Box 3: predictors of outcome of α-interferon treatment of chronic active hepatitis B

Items marked * are contraindications to therapy

	Good outcome	Poor outcome
Duration of infection	'Recent'	Congenital
Age	<40	>40
Sex	Female	Male
Ethnic origin	Non-oriental	Oriental
Sexual orientation (males)	Heterosexual	Homosexual
HIV status	Negative	Symptomatic positive
IV drug abuse	Controlled	Continued
Clinic compliance	Good	Poor*
Clinical liver disease	No decompensation	Any decompensation*
Transaminases	2–6 × normal	<2 or >6 × normal
Liver histology	Piecemeal necrosis	More than minimal fibrosis or cirrhosis*
HBV–DNA	Low	High

Case 12

An HIV-positive man with prolonged fever

History

A 34-year-old man was admitted in early 1989 for investigation of pyrexia and night sweats of 6 weeks' duration. He was known to have been HIV-positive for 5 years and had been treated for recurrent genital herpes simplex infections and genital warts. Six months before this admission he had been started on oral fluconazole 50 mg twice a week to prevent frequent recurrences of pharyngeal candidiasis. At the same time, he had started to take zidovudine 200 mg tid, and cotrimoxazole, 2 tablets daily. Apart from profuse night sweats and documented fever up to 38°C during the 6 weeks before admission, he had no significant complaints. He had drunk alcohol to excess until 6 months before this presentation but had never injected drugs.

Examination revealed a well-looking man with abnormalities of the toe nails (**1**). His temperature was 36.8°C on admission but rose to 38.2°C that night. His chest was clear, his heart sounds were normal, and his pulse was 80, with blood pressure of 165/80. His liver edge was palpable 3 cm below the costal margin and was slightly tender, and his spleen was palpable 2 cm below the costal margin. A detailed biochemical profile 4 weeks earlier had shown mild elevation of AST (52 u/l) and alkaline phosphatase (140 u/l), unchanged from 6 months previously. Investigations available the day after admission revealed:

Haematology:	Hb 11.7 g/dl
	MCV 119 fl
	WBC 2.4×10^9/l
	Neutrophils 77%, lymphocytes 15% (CD4 20×10^6/l), monocytes 7%
Biochemistry:	Urea and electrolytes normal
	Bilirubin 19 μmol/l
	AST 98 u/l
	Alk. phos. 472 u/l
Microbiology:	Urine microscopy and culture normal
	Blood cultures – no growth at 24 hours
	CSF (opening pressure 18 cm water) clear and colourless
	Lymphocytes 10×10^6/l, RBCs $<1 \times 10^6$/l
	Protein 0.63 g/l
	Glucose 2.4 mmol/l (blood glucose 4.0 mmol/l)
	Gram stain: illustrated opposite (**2**)
Imaging:	Chest x-ray: clear
	Abdominal ultrasound: non-specific diffuse changes compatible with fatty infiltration

Questions
1 What is the diagnosis?
2 What other investigations should be performed?
3 How would you manage him?

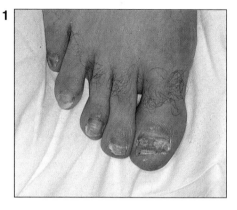

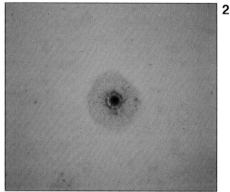

1 Toes on admission.

2 Gram stain of CSF (high power).

Answers

1 Pyrexia of unknown origin in a patient with HIV and a CD4 count <50 ×
10^6/l has a wide differential diagnosis in the absence of an immediately
obvious focal bacterial cause. Atypical *Pneumocystis carinii* infection must
always be excluded, along with CMV infection, extrapulmonary tuberculosis,
disseminated *Mycobacterium avium* complex infection (MAC), toxoplasmosis,
lymphoma and occult fungal infections. The CSF contains a yeast with a
surrounding halo due to the large capsule, and suggests cryptococcal
infection. Cryptococcal meningitis is less common in Britain than in
Australia, the USA or parts of the tropics, but can present with insidious onset
and little or no headache – as in this case.
2 The morphology of the organism is shown more readily by India ink
staining (**3**), which should be performed on all such CSF samples,
irrespective of cell content or biochemical results – which may be normal or
minimally disturbed, as in this patient. Culture of the CSF yielded *Cryptococcus
neoformans* var. *neoformans* after 5 days, sensitive to fluconazole, amphotericin,
and 5-flucytosine. Ziehl–Neelsen stains and prolonged culture of the CSF
were negative. Blood cultures were sterile after prolonged incubation. CSF
cryptococcal antigen assay was weakly positive (1:4) and serum cryptococcal
antigen titres were strongly positive (1:20,000). Retrospective assay of serum
stored 2 weeks before the onset of the patient's symptoms showed no
detectable cryptococcal antigen. Toxoplasma serology suggested past
exposure and was unchanged, and cultures of blood and urine (for CMV),
and blood and faeces (for MAC), were negative. Percutaneous liver biopsy
showed fatty change and extensive granulomata, containing numerous yeast-
like organisms (**4**, **5**). There were distinguished microscopically from

Case 12

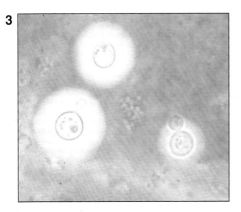

3 India ink stain of Cryptococcus neoformans in CSF sediment.

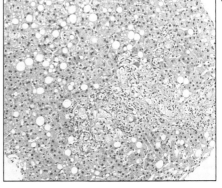

4 Liver biopsy, showing pale granulomata and fatty change.

Candida sp. and *Blastomyces* sp. by size and by selective staining of the capsule with mucicarmine. Culture of the biopsies yielded *Cryptococcus neoformans*. Scrapings from the toe nails yielded *Trichophyton interdigitale,* a common dermatophyte.

3   Amphotericin B remains the induction treatment of choice for disseminated cryptococcosis and was given intravenously for 4 weeks (total dose 1.5 g). This was complicated by transient renal failure and thrombocytopenia. Repeat cultures of CSF and of urine obtained after prostatic massage were negative at the end of the patient's induction therapy. He was subsequently maintained on oral fluconazole 200 mg daily, which was well tolerated. There was a transient rise in serum cryptococcal antigen titres to 1:80,000 at 1 month, with a slow fall over the next 12 months to 1:200. His nail infection was controlled with topical tioconazole paint.

Progress

He remained remarkably well over the following 18 months but discontinued zidovudine due to progressive pancytopenia and myopathy. Cotrimoxazole prophylaxis was changed to monthly nebulised pentamidine, and he subsequently presented with severe bilateral granulomatous *P. carinii* pneumonia, complicated by pneumothorax (**6**). This was successfully treated with high-dose intravenous cotrimoxazole. Two years later he returned with a 2-month history of cough productive of brown-coloured sputum, not responding to oral antibiotics. His general health had deteriorated with a weight loss of 4 kg and non-specific malaise. His chest x-ray (**7**) and sputum culture (**8, 9**) are shown opposite.

Questions

4   What is the likely diagnosis?
5   How should he be managed?
6   What is the prognosis?

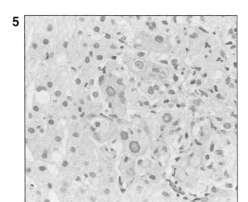

5 High-power view of liver granuloma, showing selective staining of crypto-coccus capsule with mucicarmine.

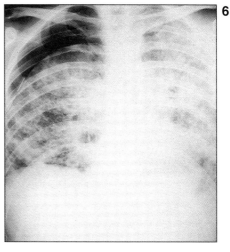

6 Chest x-ray 18 months later, showing severe bilateral granulomatous PCP with spontaneous right pneumothorax.

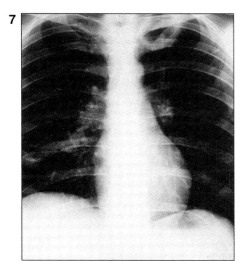

7 Chest x-ray 2 years after that shown in Figure **6**.

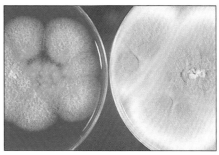

8 Subculture of sputum on blood agar (left) and Sabouraud's medium (right) after 7 days' culture.

9 Lactophenol-cotton blue stain of culture in Figure **8**.

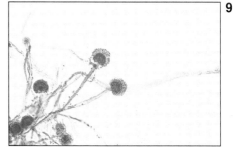

Case 12

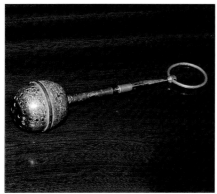

10 An aspergillum, used in the Roman Catholic church to sprinkle holy water.

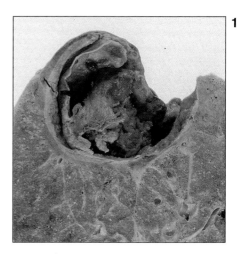

11 Left lung at autopsy, showing apical aspergilloma 4 cm in diameter.

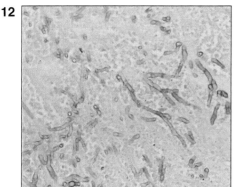

12 Invasion of tissue by aspergillus with typical dichotomous branching of septate hyphae at 45° angle (haematoxylin & eosin).

Answers

4 The chest x-ray (**7**) shows a cavity in the left upper lobe, suggesting an aspergilloma developing in the previously damaged lung. The more diffuse shadow in the right mid-zone could be due to aspergillosis or mycobacterial infection. Successive sputum samples contained fungal hyphae and the culture plates show the typical colonial appearance of *Aspergillus fumigatus*. This was confirmed by the morphology of the conidiospores shown in the lactophenol-cotton blue stain, resembling an aspergillum (**10**).

5 The ideal management would have been intravenous amphotericin B, but the patient refused this. Fluconazole has no activity against *Aspergillus* sp. and was replaced with oral itraconazole 200 mg twice daily. Serum levels of itraconazole were low and he was subsequently maintained on 600 mg daily.

6 The prognosis is usually very poor, but this patient stabilised for a further 5 months with slight improvement in his chest x-ray, despite continued positive sputum cultures for *Aspergillus* sp. He died of bronchopneumonia 4 years after his first AIDS-defining illness. Autopsy confirmed the presence of an aspergilloma in the apex of the left lung (**11**, **12**), with smaller fungal abscesses in the right lung.

Case 13

A jaundiced farmer

History

A 44-year-old Welsh farmer was admitted to a surgical ward following the sudden onset of severe colicky upper abdominal pain 4 hours previously. The pain radiated to his back but was not associated with nausea, vomiting or diarrhoea. He was well until the onset of pain, but remembered a similar but less severe episode of pain 1 month beforehand which had resolved spontaneously. He smoked 15 cigarettes a day but drank very little alcohol. He had not travelled outside north Wales.

Examination revealed a jaundiced man in obvious discomfort but with a normal temperature of 36.8°C, pulse of 90 and blood pressure of 130/80. There was tenderness in the right upper abdominal quadrant and epigastrium but he had no other abnormal physical signs. Investigations revealed:

Haematology: Hb 14.1 g/dl
WBC 13 × 10⁹/l
Neutrophils 78%, lymphocytes 24%, eosinophils 3%
ESR 7 mm/hr

Biochemistry: Urea and electrolytes normal
Bilirubin 67 μmol/l
Alk. phos. 454 u/L, ALT 337 u/l, γGT 572 u/l
Albumin 40 g/l, total protein 75 g/l

Imaging: Chest x-ray normal
Abdominal ultrasound illustrated below (**1, 2**)

Questions

1 What is the differential diagnosis?
2 What further investigations might help?
3 How should he be managed?

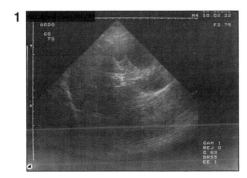
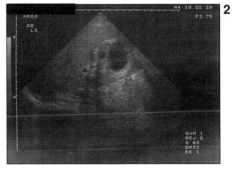

61

Case 13

Answers

1 The clinical and biochemical findings suggest cholelithiasis or another cause of acute obstruction of the biliary tree. The ultrasound pictures show a multiloculated lesion in the liver adjacent to the gall bladder, which does not contain stones. High-density echoes in the rim of this lesion indicate the presence of calcification. The multiloculated appearance suggests a hydatid cyst, although the sonographic differential diagnosis includes polycystic disease and tumours. In an endemic area of the tropics, complex shadows from a hepatoma might be confused with this. A unilocular cyst may be mistaken for a liver abscess, with the potentially disastrous consequences of anaphylaxis if a needle is introduced for diagnostic aspiration. Hydatid disease in Britain and most parts of the tropics is usually caused by the dog tapeworm, *Echinococcus granulosus.* Alveolar hydatid disease (*E. multilocularis*) is more prevalent in southern and eastern Europe, China and Alaska, and causes more diffuse tissue invasion.

2 The normal eosinophil count does not exclude the diagnosis, as eosinophilia is only found in about 15% of cases of hydatid disease. The most useful investigation is a CT scan of the abdomen (3), which here confirmed the ultrasound findings and excluded the presence of other cysts elsewhere in the abdomen or lower chest. A variety of serological tests have been employed for diagnosis. An in-house ELISA test, using crude antigen from viable hydatid cyst fluid, was strongly positive in this patient, with a positive CFT (same antigen) of 1:64. The Casoni skin test cross-reacts with other trematodes and helminths, and is obsolete.

3 Hydatid cysts most commonly affect the liver (70%) and the lung (20%), with cysts at more than one location in about 20% of patients. They are frequently asymptomatic and heavy calcification visible on plain abdominal x-rays usually indicates a parasitologically inert cyst. The natural history of such cysts is unknown, but surgery is probably only necessary if cysts cause local or systemic symptoms due to pressure effects. This patient's jaundice could have been due to local pressure on the biliary tree, but is more likely to have been caused by temporary biliary obstruction by the passage of daughter cysts via a communication between the cyst and the biliary tree. This occurs in about 15% of symptomatic liver cysts and can be diagnosed and relieved by endoscopic retrograde pancreatography (ERCP) with peroperative removal of obstructing material. Patients with lung cysts typically present with a cough and haemoptysis, including expectoration of cyst membrane. Rarely, patients with rapidly growing hepatic or multiple intra-abdominal cysts present with cachexia and features suggesting carcinoma. This is more common with alveolar hydatids. Anaphylaxis due to rupture of cysts, either spontaneously or after trauma, is unusual.

This patient's acute symptoms resolved spontaneously over 5 days and his liver-function tests returned to normal. He was given a trial of oral albendazole therapy in 3 cycles each of 400 mg (10 mg/kg/day) bid for 28 days followed by a 'drug holiday' for 14 days. Albendazole therapy results in resolution of cysts in about only 25% of cases, with improvement in a further 50%. It is most useful for therapy of thin-walled abdominal cysts or for controlling inoperable disease, but is less likely to be effective in patients with calcified cysts. Praziquantel (50 mg/kg/day for 14 days) is still being

3 Contrast-enhanced CT scan of patient, showing daughter cysts within solitary calcified hepatic cyst adjacent to the gallbladder.

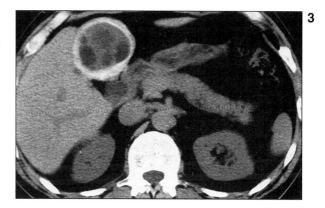

3

4

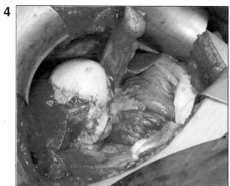

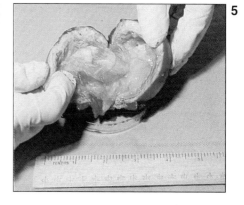

5

4 Laparotomy revealed the cyst (white) adhering to the gallbladder.

5 The removed cyst, opened to show thick wall and degenerate contents.

6 Low-power view (polarised light) of cyst contents reveals numerous hooklets, which are strongly birefringent.

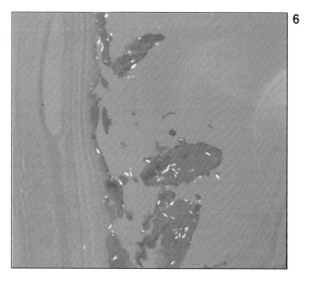

6

Case 13

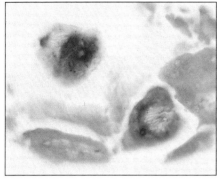 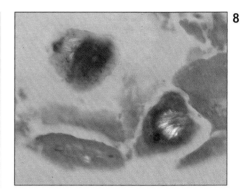

7 High-power view of degenerate protoscolex in cyst debris (haematoxylin & eosin).

8 View of same field as **7** in polarised light shows hooklets more clearly.

evaluated. Either of these agents can be used perioperatively to sterilise protoscolices spilt during surgery. Serial scans showed minimal disruption of the internal structure of the cyst, and the patient continued to experience intermittent right hypochondrial pain. Six months after his initial presentation the cyst was removed intact with subsegmental hepatectomy and cholecystectomy (**4–8**). Three months after the operation his serum hydatid ELISA was more strongly positive but the CFT titre had not changed. An initial rise in either test sometimes occurs after operation and serological tests are unreliable for monitoring the success of treatment.

A young man with stroke

History

A 36-year-old man was admitted to hospital following the sudden onset of left-sided weakness. For 7 days prior to admission he had been troubled by diffuse musculoskeletal pains, headache and sweats, which had been attributed to influenza by his general practitioner, who had prescribed aspirin and co-amoxyclav 375 mg 8 hourly.

On examination his temperature was 38.9°C and pulse 96, with blood pressure of 150/70. Lesions were present on his fingers (1), and there was a soft early diastolic murmur at the left sternal edge. On neurological examination he had a dense left hemiparesis.

Haematology:	Hb 13.4 g/dl
	WBC 8.4 × 10⁹/l
	Neutrophils 88%, lymphocytes 10%
Biochemistry:	Na 135 mmol/l
	K 4.8 mmol/l
	Urea 10 mmol/l
	Creatinine 130 μmol/l
	Bilirubin 27 μmol/l
	Alk. phos. 130 u/l
	AST 52 u/l

Urine microscopy: WBC 10×10^6/l, RBC 30×10^6/l

Questions

1 What are the finger lesions and what is the most likely diagnosis?
2 What is the likely cause of the hemiparesis?
3 What abnormality does the ECG (2) show and how might this be relevant?
4 What investigations would you regard as most important at this stage?
5 What treatment would you start?
6 Would you anticoagulate this patient?

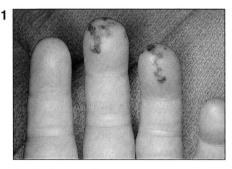

1 Lesions on fingers.

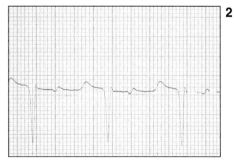

2 ECG on admission (lead V₁).

Case 14

Answers

1   These are embolic lesions, suggestive of infective endocarditis (IE). The brief history and florid nature of the lesions suggests a staphylococcal aetiology. Despite careful history and examination, no portal of entry could be defined.

2   He has had an embolism to the right middle cerebral artery. Neurological events are a presenting feature in about 20% of patients with endocarditis. Any patient who presents with a stroke and who has no underlying risk factors for cerebrovascular disease must be carefully evaluated for possible endocarditis.

3   The ECG shows first-degree block (PR interval 0.24 seconds). While this may be a normal variant, it suggests extension of infection beyond the valve ring into the atrio-ventricular conducting system.

4 and 5   The most critical investigation is to obtain blood for culture. The recent oral antimicrobials may render blood cultures negative for up to 2 weeks; ideally, all antimicrobials should be discontinued and blood cultures taken regularly while the patient is closely observed. This problem may be partially circumvented by taking blood into bottles containing antimicrobial absorbing resin (3). However, treatment should be started without delay in a patient such as this one, with strong evidence of endocarditis.

Three sets of cultures taken by separate venepunctures must be collected and intravenous antimicrobials should be commenced afterwards to cover the major bacterial causes of IE, *Staphylococcus aureus*, viridans streptococci and *Enterococcus* sp. A typical initial combination would be ampicillin 12 g/day and flucloxacillin 12 g/day in divided doses, with gentamicin in a modest dose – yielding peak blood levels of 3–5 mg/l, which is sufficient to provide synergistic activity against streptococci. This must be modified subsequently in the light of the results of cultures and sensitivity tests, including estimates of the MIC and MBC of antibiotics for the organism. These are essential to determine the required nature and duration of chemotherapy.

Echocardiography is helpful in assessing whether the infection extends to the valve ring or myocardium, the size of vegetations and the degree of valvular dysfunction, and hence the potential need for surgical intervention (Box 1). An echocardiogram showing no evidence of valvular vegetations does not, however, exclude infective endocarditis – even when performed by

Box 1: indications for surgery in left-sided infective endocarditis	
Definite indications:	Moderate-to-severe congestive cardiac failure Valvular obstruction Valve ring or myocardial abscess Persistent bacteraemia (more than one week on adequate treatment) Fungal endocarditis
Relative indications:	Difficult-to-treat organisms, e.g. staphylococci and Gram negatives Presence of vegetations on echocardiography Emboli

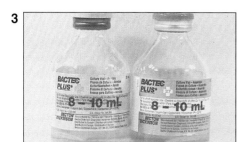

3 Blood culture bottles containing resin to absorb antimicrobials.

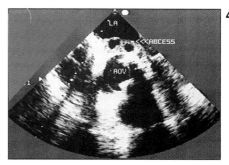

4 Transoesophageal echocardiogram from another patient, showing small vegetation on aortic valve (AOV) and abscess in aortic valve root.

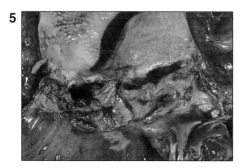

5 Vegetations on aortic valve.

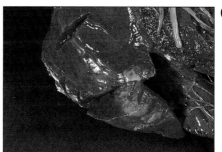

6 Abscess in left ventricle.

the transoesophageal technique, which is more sensitive than conventional transthoracic scans (**4**).

6   Emboli secondary to IE are not generally regarded as an indication for anticoagulation. The risk of embolism falls as soon as effective antimicrobial treatment has been started.

Progress
The patient started a course of antimicrobials after three sets of blood cultures had been taken as outlined above. The next evening four of the six bottles had grown Gram-positive cocci in clusters, which on sub-culture were identified as *S. aureus*. The fever persisted and his general condition rapidly deteriorated. An echocardiogram showed aortic valve vegetations and significant aortic incompetence. While being prepared for aortic valve replacement he had a further cerebral embolism, resulting in a right hemiparesis, and he died later that day.

At autopsy the major findings were acute endocarditis of the aortic valve (**5**) and a myocardial abscess (**6**) with septic emboli in the cerebral arteries.

The unconscious grandmother

History

A 64-year-old woman was brought to the emergency room late on a Saturday night in February after her daughter had found her unconscious at home. She had complained of vague chest pains, malaise and a productive cough for 7 days but this had been improving when her daughter saw her 24 hours before admission. She had no significant previous medical history despite smoking 30 cigarettes a day. She lived alone but had frequent contact with her two daughters and regularly looked after her two grandchildren aged 7 and 8, one of whom had recently had a respiratory illness.

On arrival at the hospital she was extremely ill with an obvious rash (1–3), a stiff neck, and central cyanosis breathing room air. Her temperature was 38.5°C, pulse 150 in atrial fibrillation, blood pressure was 110/75 and respiratory rate 30. She was moaning and rolling around, and was unable to speak coherently, obey commands or withdraw her limbs from painful stimuli. Her pupils reacted equally to light and there was possible early papilloedema on fundoscopy. There were no focal neurological signs apart from an upgoing left plantar response. The heart sounds were normal, central venous pressure was not clinically raised, and her extremities were warm – but there were scattered fine inspiratory crackles in both lung fields. She was rapidly transferred to the ITU, where she required sedation and intubation. Investigations taken in the emergency room showed:

Haematology:	Hb 10.6 g/dl
	WBC 25.5×10^9/l
	Neutrophils 90%
	Platelets 125×10^9/l
	Prothrombin time 18 secs (INR 1.5), APTT 37.1 secs
	(control 35.3)
Biochemistry:	Na 137 mmol/l
	K 3.4 mmol/l
	Urea 8.9 mmol/l
	Glucose 6.7 mmol/l
	Albumin 32 g/l
Blood gases:	pH 7.46, pO_2 8.1 KPa (61 mmHg), pCO_2 4.2 KPa (32
(room air)	mmHg)
(40% oxygen)	pH 7.48, pO_2 19.2 KPa (144 mmHg), pCO_2 4.7 KPa (35
	mmHg)
Sputum	
microscopy:	Illustrated opposite (4)
Radiology:	Possible right upper lobe consolidation and bibasal Kerley B
	lines without cardiomegaly (not shown)

Questions

1 What is the differential diagnosis?
2 How would you interpret the sputum microscopy?
3 What are the essential aspects of immediate management and investigation?
4 What advice should be given to her contacts?

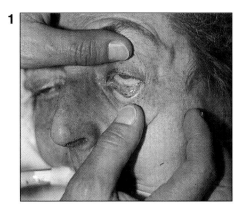

1 Subconjunctival rash.

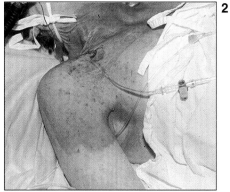

2 Rash on trunk and upper arm.

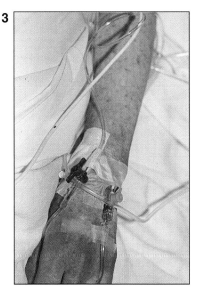

3 Rash on arm and dusky hue of hand.

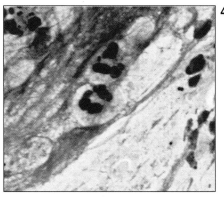

4 Gram stain (under decolourised) of sputum obtained in emergency room.

Case 15

Answers

1   The most likely diagnosis is meningococcal meningitis and septicaemia. The physical signs on admission satisfy current criteria for defining the sepsis syndrome: that is, clinical evidence of infection plus tachypnoea (>20 breaths/min), tachycardia (>90) and hyperthermia (>38.4°C), together with acute alteration in mental status. A similar clinical picture may accompany bacteraemia caused by many Gram-positive and Gram-negative organisms. In this case, pneumococcal septicaemia and listeriosis were considered, and staphylococcal septicaemia complicating influenza was included in the differential diagnosis – although there were no specific features of this on the chest x-ray. She was admitted during an influenza A epidemic and invasive meningococcal disease is more likely to occur in smokers or following viral respiratory infections that damage the respiratory epithelium. Rarely, invasive meningococcal disease presents with predominantly lower respiratory symptoms due to meningococcal pneumonia. There were no signs of endocarditis and her atrial fibrillation was thought to be a toxic manifestion of sepsis, although it raised the possibility of an underlying lung neoplasm.

2   The sputum microcopy shows Gram-negative diplococci within neutrophils. These could be either *Moraxella catarrhalis* or *Neisseria* sp., which cannot be distinguished morphologically on the Gram stain. Cultures of sputum and of blood taken in the emergency room yielded *N. meningitidis* Group B within 24 hours.

3   Initial management should include protection of the airway, breathing and circulation (see 'Progress and outcome' opposite). In this clinical situation antimicrobial agents should be given without delay and the emergency room doctor correctly gave intravenous benzyl penicillin 2.4 g immediately after taking blood for culture and establishing intravenous access. The antibiotics were changed to cefotaxime and erythromycin (to cover atypical respiratory pathogens) on transfer to ITU. Metronidazole was given to cover the remote possibility of anaerobic brain abscess. This woman had several features contraindicating lumbar puncture: that is, sepsis syndrome, possible papilloedema, and a focal neurological sign. Empirical treatment should be instituted and altered according to subsequent results of CT scan, CSF and other cultures. Although Gram stain and culture of material from skin lesions occasionally yields organisms in meningococcal disease, this was not successful. The therapeutic role of steroids has not been established for the treatment of adults with bacterial meningitis. Adrenal haemorrhage in the Waterhouse–Friderichsen syndrome (**5**) is usually accompanied by raised levels of serum cortisol and is not an indication for steroid therapy.

4   Close family and 'kissing contacts' should be given chemoprophylaxis as soon as possible to reduce the remote risk of developing invasive meningococcal disease. Chemoprophylaxis should be given as soon as the clinical diagnosis has been made for the index case and should not await culture results or results of pretreatment throat swabs from contacts (which need not be taken).

Currently recommended agents for meningococcal chemoprophylaxis include rifampicin 600 mg bid for 48 hours (10 mg/kg bid for children) or

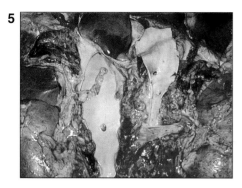

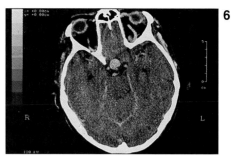

5 Bilateral adrenal haemorrhage in a young man who died 12 hours after first symptoms of meningococcal sepsis.

6 Contrast-enhanced CT scan of head 18 hours after admission, showing high attenuation rounded area filling the pituitary fossa but no blood in the subarachnoid space.

ciprofloxacin 500 mg in a single dose. Ceftriaxone (1 g single dose) has also been shown to be effective in epidemic situations and is the drug of choice for pregnant contacts. Sulphadiazine cannot be used for sporadic cases because of the high rate of primary resistance, subsequently confirmed in this case (MIC 32 mg/l). Administration of chemoprophylaxis is difficult to co-ordinate, especially if patients are admitted outside routine working hours. The public health authorities should be notified immediately of the details of the case to enable them to follow up contacts in the community. Our practice is to prescribe for contacts who accompany the patient to hospital – this means that hospital staff in areas likely to receive patients with meningococcal disease should have immediate access to local policy guidelines and that supplies of appropriate antibiotics should be readily available.

Vaccines are now available for *N. mengitidis* Groups A and C but are not used in the UK for 'blind' immunisation of contacts because the majority of sporadic cases are caused by Group B organisms. Policies for chemoprophylaxis and immunisation of contacts of a single sporadic case in institutions such as schools are still under debate.

Progress and outcome

The patient's condition rapidly deteriorated with hypotension and oliguria requiring dopamine and dobutamine, and she developed mild adult respiratory distress syndrome. Her condition was not stable enough for a CT scan to be performed until 18 hours after admission. This suggested that she had suffered a pituitary haemorrhage (**6**), and so intravenous hydrocortisone therapy was added. The atrial fibrillation responded to short-term digoxin therapy. She was ventilated for 14 days and left hospital after a total of 5 weeks. Subsequent pituitary function tests were normal and CT scans showed resolution of the pituitary haemorrhage. Serological tests confirmed that she had influenza A at the time of admission. She had no apparent neurological deficit at review 3 months after admission, but was re-admitted a month later following a right frontal lobe infarct.

Atypical chest and abdominal pain

History

A 65-year-old retired sailor is admitted to a surgical ward following the sudden onset of continuous intrascapular back pain 2 days beforehand, associated with epigastric pain. He has been anorexic for 1 year with 15 kg weight loss. He admits to drinking 6 pints of beer every night with additional whisky and to smoking up to 100 cigarettes a day, but he has not been vomiting or coughing. His past history includes non-insulin dependent diabetes and a small stroke 7 years earlier, and he is taking indomethacin for osteoarthritis of the knees.

He is unwell and sweaty, with a temperature of 38˚C, pulse of 90, blood pressure of 140/90 and a respiratory rate of 20. No focal chest signs are detected. His liver is slightly enlarged and tender, and his spleen is palpable. His ECG shows sinus tachycardia without ischaemic changes.

Haematology:	Hb 15.6 g/dl
	MCV 108 fl
	WBC 17.4×10^9/l
	Neutrophils 86% with marked left shift and 3% metamyelocytes
	Platelets 136×10^9/l
Biochemistry:	Na 126 mmol/l
	K 4.6 mmol/l
	Urea 5.7 mmol/l
	Glucose 15.5 mmol/l
	Amylase 34 u/l
	Bilirubin 41 μmol/l
	Alk. phos. 96 u/l
	AST 7 u/l
	γGT 114 u/l
	Albumin 29 g/l, total protein 60 g/l
Imaging:	Thoracic spine x-rays: normal
	Abdominal ultrasound: splenomegaly, no ascites or biliary obstruction
	Chest x-ray: illustrated opposite (1)

The differential diagnosis is thought to be either pancreatitis, a peptic ulcer secondary to indomethacin, or upper gastrointestinal neoplasm, all superimposed on alcoholic cirrhosis. Over the next 3 days he becomes desperately ill with progressive jaundice, falling blood pressure and poor peripheral perfusion, and he is transferred to ITU. His arterial pO_2 while breathing room air falls to 6.46 kPa (48 mmHg) and a further chest x-ray shows a worsening picture (2). He is given ampicillin, and a diagnostic tap of 100 ml of serosanguinous fluid taken from the right chest is sent for

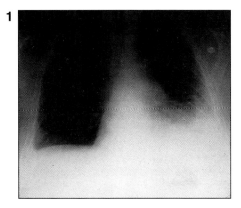

1 Chest x-ray on admission (day 1).

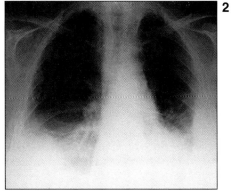

2 Chest x-ray on day 4.

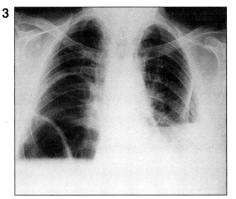

3 Chest x-ray on day 7.

4 Gram stain of fluid aspirated from left chest on day 7.

biochemical analysis, which reveals a protein content of 33 g/l and normal amylase of 98 u/l. Three days later he is more dyspnoeic and has signs of hepatic failure. The repeat chest x-ray is illustrated (3). Chocolate-coloured fluid is aspirated from his left chest and sent for microbiological examination (4–6).

Questions

1 What does the chest x-ray series illustrate?
2 How would you interpret the Gram stain and culture results, and what is their diagnostic significance?
3 What antimicrobial therapy would you recommend?
4 What further investigations and management are indicated?

Case 16

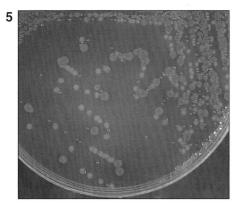 5

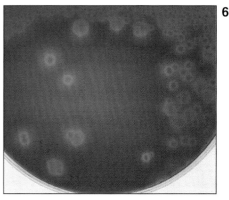 6

5 Aerobic culture of the pleural aspirate on blood agar.

6 Anerobic culture of the pleural aspirate on blood agar with kanamycin added to suppress coliforms.

Answers

1 The chest x-ray on admission shows a moderate left pleural effusion and a small right pleural effusion, without pneumothorax. The second radiograph shows an increase in size of both effusions, which have become encysted. The third x-ray shows loculated gas and a hydropneumothorax on the right, and a loculated cavity and effusion on the left.

2 The Gram stain reveals mixed flora, including large Gram-positive rods, Gram-positive cocci, and pleomorphic Gram-negative rods. The cultures show a mixed growth, including coliforms and streptococci, with *Clostridium* sp. visible on the anaerobic plate to which kanamycin has been added to suppress the growth of facultative anaerobes. This is compatible with bowel flora and in this context is diagnostic of oesophageal rupture (Boerhaave's syndrome).

3 His antibiotic therapy was changed to cefotaxime and metronidazole, to cover Gram-positive and Gram-negative organisms and the high likelihood of penicillin-resistant anaerobic infection. Alternative suitable regimens could include imipenem, or combination therapy with benzyl penicillin, metronidazole and an aminoglycoside or aztreonam. While empirical antifungal treatment is not usually required at this stage, the risk of superinfection with yeasts is high and close bacteriological monitoring is essential.

4 The most critical aspect of management is drainage of the empyemas. He was too ill for surgical drainage, but wide-bore chest drains were inserted, yielding a large volume of air and fluid from both sides of the chest. Gastrograffin swallow (**7**, **8**) confirmed the presence of an oesophageal tear in an unusually high position. The more typical radiographic picture of such a tear is illustrated in Figure **9**.

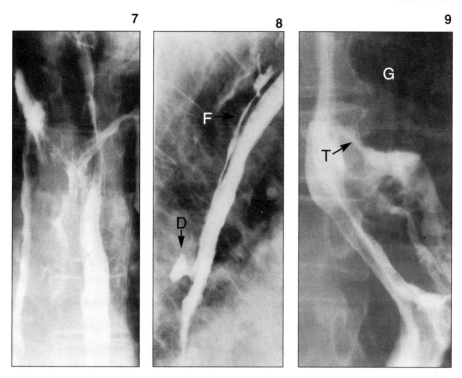

7, 8 Gastrograffin swallow, showing a high leak of gastrograffin which is travelling down both sides of the posterior mediastinum in the a–p view. The lateral view (**8**) reveals a fistulous track (F) posterior to the oesophagus and a leak or diverticulum (D) in the lower third of the oesophagus.

9 Gastrograffin swallow from a different patient, showing the more usual position of tears at the junction of the upper two-thirds and lower third of the oesophagus (T), with free gas in the mediastinum (G).

Progress

Oesophagoscopy confirmed the presence of a posterior oesophageal tear, which was managed conservatively by nasogastric tube-feeding in view of the patient's poor general condition. Antibiotic treatment and continuous drainage led to considerable resolution of the empyemas over the next month and repeat gastrograffin swallows suggested that the oesophageal tear had healed. However, his condition deteriorated and he eventually died with hepatic failure 3 months after admission despite formal surgical drainage of his chest. The postmortem confirmed the presence of cirrhosis with splenomegaly and showed a persisting high oesophageal tear 2.5 cm long. This case illustrates many of the problems encountered in the management of empyema, including delayed recognition, the necessity for culturing all pleural fluid aspirates, and the need for an aggressive surgical approach.

A painful blistering rash

History

A 56-year-old builder, previously in good health, is admitted to an orthopaedic ward with a 24-hour history of pain in the right hip and buttock associated with diffuse myalgia, headache and fever. On examination his temperature is 37.5°C, pulse 90 and blood pressure is 130/75. There is an area of tenderness over the right buttock but there are no visible skin changes nor any pain on hip movement. Baseline laboratory tests reveal a marked leucocytosis (total WBC count 25.9 × 10⁹/l), with 95% polymorphonuclear cells. Radiographs of the chest and hips are normal. Blood cultures are taken and intravenous cefuroxime 750 mg 8 hourly is started for suspected septic arthritis. The next day he collapses with a pulse of 150 and an unrecordable blood pressure, and an extensive area of blistering skin rash has appeared, extending from his initial area of pain across the back and down the right leg (1).

Haematology:	Hb 12.3 g/dl
	WBC 31.5 × 10⁹/l
	Neutrophils 98% with marked left shift
	Platelets 215 × 10⁹/l
Biochemistry:	Na 133 mmol/l
	K 5.3 mmol/l
	Urea 14.3 mmol/l
	Creatinine 187 µmol/l
	Glucose 1.9 mmol/l
	Bilirubin 22 µmol/l
	Alk. phos. 172 u/l
	ALT 35 u/l
	Prothrombin time 19.5 secs (INR 1.4), APTT 50 secs (control 28.5 secs)
	CK 1176 u/l (100% MM isoenzyme)
Blood gases: (room air)	pO$_2$ 8.4 kPa (63 mmHg), pCO$_2$ 7.3 kPa (55 mmHg)
Radiology:	Chest x-ray illustrated opposite (2)
ECG:	Normal
Microbiology:	Gram stain (3) and subculture (4) of initial blood culture opposite

Questions

1 What immediate steps would you take at this stage?
2 What do the Gram stain and subculture of the blood culture isolate show?
3 What is the most likely identity of the blood isolate in view of the clinical progress?
4 Are the biochemical changes compatible with non-specific manifestations of sepsis or should other diagnoses be considered?

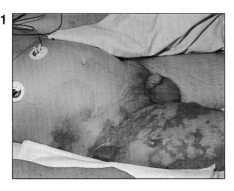

1 Rash on second day of admission.

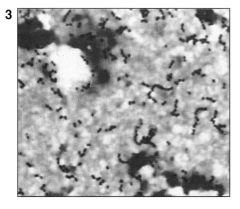

2 Chest x-ray on second day of admission.

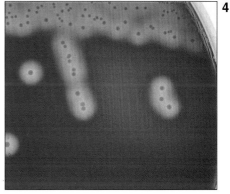

3 Gram stain of blood culture isolate at 24 hours.

4 Subculture of blood isolate after overnight anaerobic incubation on blood agar.

Case 17

5

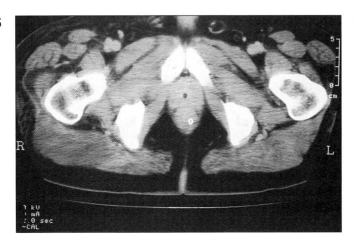

5 CT scan through the pelvis, showing oedema of skin, underlying soft tissue and muscle.

Answers

1   This patient has profound shock and a chest x-ray suggestive of adult respiratory distress syndrome. He needs aggressive resuscitation with intravascular fluids, inotropes, and respiratory support.

2   Long chains of Gram-positive cocci are present in the Gram stain and the subculture shows a clear zone of β-haemolysis around each colony.

3   In the context of the sudden onset of shock, Lancefield group A β–haemolytic streptococci, which elaborate a range of potent exotoxins, are most probable.

4   The slight increase in bilirubin and rise in alkaline phosphatase are common non-specific features of sepsis. The low blood glucose is a relatively uncommon but recognised feature of severe sepsis. The very high CK of skeletal muscle origin is suggestive of rhabdomyolysis, in this case due to localised streptococcal myositis. This is illustrated in the CT scan (**5**).

Despite high-dose benzyl penicillin (1.8 g 6 hourly), inotrope support and ventilation in ITU, the patient became oliguric and required haemodialysis. Debridement of the necrotic skin down to deep fascia failed to improve the manifestations of systemic sepsis and he died 10 days after admission.

Group A streptococci associated with severe toxic shock appear to have become more common recently in both the USA and Europe. The presentation with severe pain out of proportion to the initial physical signs is characteristic of this syndrome. While the nature of the toxins produced has not been fully elucidated, streptococcal pyrogenic exotoxins A, B and C may all play a role. These toxins appear to behave as superantigens, with the capacity to bind directly to the Vβ regions of T-cell receptors and hence to stimulate a much larger population of T lymphocytes than conventional antigens, which require prior processing by antigen-presenting cells. The brisk subsequent release of potent cytokines, such as TNF-α from monocytes and TNF-β from T lymphocytes, probably accounts for the rapid and often irreversible shock syndrome.

Case 18

Spot diagnosis 1

History

A 27-year-old nursery nurse is referred by her general practitioner with a 5-day history of headache, tiredness, muscle pain and vague fever. Three days ago she developed a pruritic rash on the nape of her neck, spreading to her trunk and face. She has also noticed soreness in her mouth and vulva. She is a non-smoker and has no respiratory symptoms. There is no significant medical history and she is not pregnant.

Examination reveals a well-looking woman with an obvious rash (**1**) extending to the trunk and involving the gums (**2**) and vulva. Her temperature is 37.2°C, pulse 100, blood pressure 120/80, and respiratory rate 12. Her chest is clear and the remainder of the physical examination is normal.

Haematology:	Hb 14.6 g/dl
	WBC $4.6 \times 10^9/l$
	Neutrophils 60%, lymphocytes 30%, monocytes 8%
	Platelets $128 \times 10^9/l$
Biochemistry:	Urea and electrolytes normal
	Alk. phos. 80 u/l
	AST 56 u/l
	Bilirubin 18 μmol/l
Radiology:	Chest x-ray clear

Questions

1 What is the diagnosis and how might it be confirmed?
2 What are the important complications?
3 What are the risks of this infection in pregnancy?
4 What are the infection control implications?

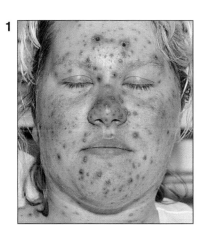

1 Patient on admission.
2 Painful lesion on gum.

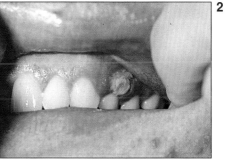

Case 18

Answers

1   This woman has chickenpox (varicella) caused by varicella zoster virus (VZV). After an incubation period of 2–3 weeks successive crops of vesicles develop which progress to scabs. The illness is characterised by the presence of vesicles in all stages of evolution, typically more central than peripheral in distribution. The diagnosis rarely needs confirmatory tests unless the presentation is atypical, when involvement of mucous membranes is a useful diagnostic feature. Mild elevation of transaminases and mild thrombocytopenia are common. Electron microscopy of vesicle fluid reveals herpes virus particles, which are distinguished from herpes simplex by culture or immunofluorescence. Serum VZV IgM antibodies rise within 7 days of the onset of the rash in immunocompetent individuals. Tzanck smears from the base of unroofed vesicles, showing multinucleated giant cells, do not distinguish varicella from other herpes viruses.

2   Chickenpox is more severe in adults. Smokers and pregnant women are particularly prone to pneumonitis (**3, 4**), typically at its worst on the 4th day after appearance of the rash. The next most frequent complication is encephalitis, which usually causes transient truncal ataxia in children. Encephalitis is less common but more generalised in adults and can result in permanent neurological deficit. Haemorrhagic complications are rare. All complications are more severe in immunocompromised individuals and neonates (**5, 6**). Herpes zoster (shingles) arises from reactivation of latent virus and is more common in the elderly and the immunosuppressed. The severity and duration of a chickenpox rash can be slightly reduced with high-dose acyclovir, but this is not usually prescribed for mild infections of immunocompetent children and adults. Immunocompromised individuals and immunocompetent adults with complicated chickenpox should receive intravenous acyclovir 10–15 mg/kg tid for 5–7 days depending on clinical response. Although acyclovir is not licensed for use in pregnancy, most physicians would prescribe it for a pregnant woman with varicella pneumonia after appropriate counselling.

3   The greatest risk to the fetus occurs if the mother develops chickenpox within 1 week before or after delivery, with a neonatal mortality of up to 30%. The risk falls over the next 3 weeks. Babies born to mothers who develop chickenpox less than 7 days before, or 28 days after, delivery should receive specific varicella zoster immune globulin (VZIG), and many physicians would give prophylactic acyclovir to a neonate born to a mother who develops a rash within 7 days before or after delivery. VZIG should also be given to infants in contact with chickenpox if born at less than 30 weeks' gestation or weighing less than 1 kg at birth, and to normal neonates in contact with chickenpox or herpes zoster if the mother has no detectable antibody. Chickenpox in early pregnancy (first 4–5 months) results in the congenital varicella syndrome in less than 1% of deliveries.

   Infection in later pregnancy predisposes the fetus to herpes zoster in early childhood. Pregnant women in contact with chickenpox should receive VZIG only if they do not have a definite history of previous chickenpox or herpes zoster, or demonstrable IgG antibodies (present in about two-thirds). This will reduce the severity of the illness but not prevent infection. Similar advice applies for immunocompromised patients. Vaccination with live attenuated organisms is effective but its use to date has been restricted mainly to children with leukaemia.

4   Nosocomial infection is a genuine hazard. Hospitalised patients with chickenpox and early herpes zoster should be nursed in isolation rooms with negative airflow control and using strict barrier precautions, preferably by staff known to be immune to chickenpox. Airborne spread to distant parts of the ward is well documented, and immunocompromised patients should not be present on the same open ward. Non-immune health care workers exposed to a case should not have contact with immunocompromised patients, neonates or pregnant women from 8–21 days after the exposure.

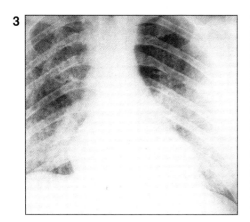

3   Chickenpox pneumonitis in a 30-year-old smoker.

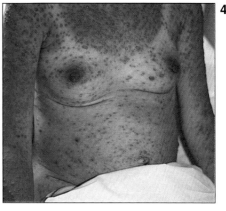

4   A pregnant woman with extensive rash, more prominent in hyperaemic areas of sunburn.

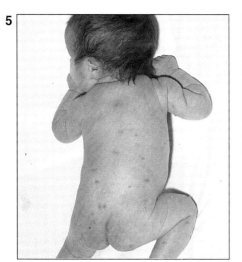

5   Perinatal chickenpox.

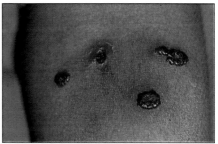

6   Haemorrhagic lesions and bleeding from venepuncture site – a boy with aplastic anaemia (platelets 20× 10⁹/l).

Case 19

Fever after bone marrow transplant

History

A 46-year-old woman developed a fever six days after autologous bone marrow transplantation for relapsed T-cell lymphoma. She had been receiving oral ciprofloxacin 500 mg bid and acyclovir 200 mg tid since the onset of neutropenia. No focus of infection was identified on clinical examination or chest radiograph and she was started on gentamicin 120 mg bid and piperacillin 4 g tid intravenously. On the eighth day she remained pyrexial despite the addition of teicoplanin 400 mg daily, for a suspected Hickman line infection, after coagulase negative staphylococci had been isolated from blood cultures taken from the line. On the tenth day post-transplant she developed a few asymmetrical, painless, papular lesions predominantly on the limbs (**1, 2**). Investigations at this time revealed:

Haematology:	Hb 10.1 g/dl
	WBC 0.1×10^9/l (100% lymphocytes)
Biochemistry:	Na 131 mmol/l
	K 4.5 mmol/l
	Urea 8.5 mmol/l
	Creatinine 135 µmol/l
	Bilirubin 22 µmol/l
	Alk. phos. 123 u/l
	AST 49 u/l
Radiology:	Serial chest x-rays are illustrated (**3, 4**)
Microbiology:	No growth after 48 hours from further blood cultures taken after addition of teicoplanin to regimen

Questions

1. What are the likely causes of the rash and how might this be confirmed?
2. What changes are shown on the chest x-ray?
3. What are the most likely causes of the continuing fever?
4. What treatment would you initiate?

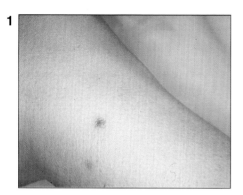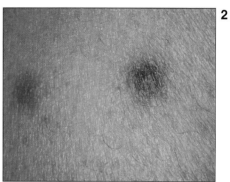

1, 2 Rash on leg on tenth post-transplant day.

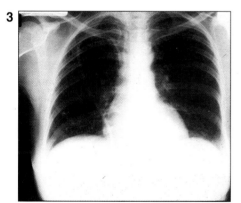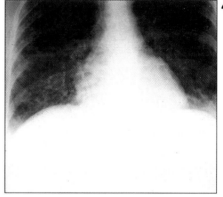

3, 4 Chest x-rays before (**3**) and 10 days after (**4**) transplant.

Case 19

Answers

1 A scanty papular rash with some lesions progressing to nodules is strongly suggestive of systemic yeast infection, especially with *Candida* sp. Bacterial infection is likely to progress more rapidly and to be associated with positive blood cultures, while failure to grow yeast from blood is not uncommon even in systemic infections. Confirmation of the nature of the rash is best made by biopsy, although a Gram stain of a fine needle aspirate may yield a more rapid result. A rash of this type may occasionally be due to drugs. Graft versus host disease would not occur at this stage post transplantation.

2 The chest x-ray shows nodular infiltrates which are suggestive of haematogenous infection rather than a primary pneumonia, and in this context should again raise the possibility that a yeast infection is present.

3 Continuing fever in a profoundly neutropenic patient who is receiving broad spectrum antimicrobials and has negative blood cultures has a wide differential diagnosis which requires careful clinical and laboratory assessment, but often defies a definite diagnosis (Box 1). Failure of comprehensive anti-bacterial treatment to control the fever after 5–7 days is regarded by many clinicians to be an indication to initiate systemic antifungal chemotherapy with amphotericin B, even in the absence of any other findings to support the diagnosis of fungal infection. This policy is embraced by the planned progressive therapy protocols for febrile neutropenic patients which are used in many units.

4 In this patient, with several features supporting this diagnosis, amphotericin B should be started immediately. Since the clinical features are suggestive of yeast rather than aspergillus infection, it would be reasonable to give a dose of 0.5 mg/kg rather than the higher dose of 1–1.5 mg/kg recommended for aspergillus infection. There is evidence that prophylaxis with very high doses of fluconazole (400 mg daily) can reduce the risk of systemic fungal infection in bone marrow transplant recipients, although it will not cover aspergillus or mucor and has been associated with a relative increase in *C. krusei* infections.

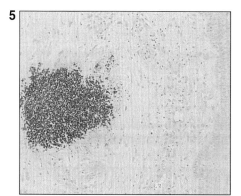 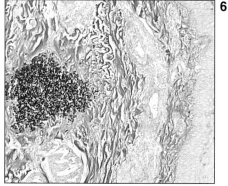

5, 6 Low power views of skin biopsy stained with PAS (**5**) and Grocott's stain (**6**).

Box 1: the assessment of the febrile neutropenic patient with continuing or recurrent fever on first-line anti-bacterial treatment

CLINICAL ASSESSMENT

Site	Symptoms/signs	Likely pathogen
Mouth	Necrotizing gingivitis Vesicles/ulcers	Anaerobic bacteria Herpes simplex
Sinuses/nose	Sinusitis/ulceration	Aspergillus sp. Mucor sp.
Oesophagus	Dysphagia (oesophagitis)	Candida sp. Herpes simplex
Lower gastrointestinal tract	Abdominal pain (typhlitis) Diarrhoea	Anaerobic bacteria Clostridium difficile
Perianal area	Tenderness/frank cellulitis Vesicles	Anaerobic bacteria Herpes simplex
IV catheter tunnel and exit site	Cellulitis	Coagulase-negative staphylococci Diphtheroids
Skin	Ecthyma gangrenosum	Pseudomonas aeruginosa
	Nodules/pustules	Yeasts
	Vesicles	Herpes simplex Varicella zoster

MICROBIOLOGICAL ASSESSMENT

Regular blood cultures via both central line and peripheral veins.
Biopsy of any accessible foci of infection for Gram stain, Grocott stain and culture.
Serial C-reactive protein measurement helpful to assess response and to rule out drug fever.
Serum for aspergillus and candida antigen assays currently a research tool.

IMAGING

Chest x-ray.
Other imaging techniques directed by clinical findings.

Progress

The skin biopsy showed yeasts in dense colonies in the dermis (**5, 6**). Despite the administration of systemic amphotericin B, the patient remained febrile, became confused and developed features of multiorgan failure. She died one week later and at post mortem widely disseminated foci of *C. albicans* were found (**7–12**).

Case 19

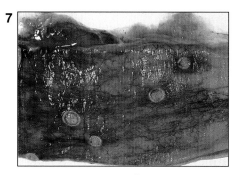

7 Oesophagus at autopsy with large candidal ulcers.

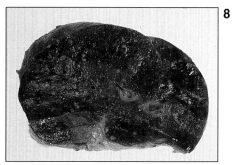

8 Cut section of spleen with 'miliary' nodules of C. albicans.

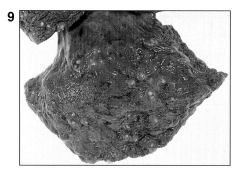

9 Lung with plueral nodules.

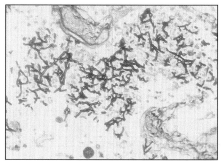

10 Pseudohyphae of C. albicans in lung tissue (high power, Grocott).

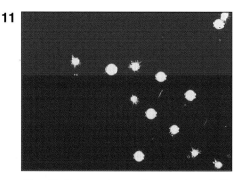

11 Stellate and smooth colonies of C. albicans on blood agar after aerobic incubation for 48 hours.

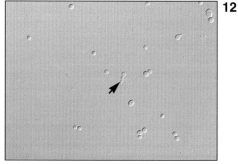

12 C. albicans producing a germ tube (arrow) after two hours incubation in serum (Nomarski).

Case 20

Severe pneumonia

History

A 67-year-old man with a history of ischaemic heart disease was admitted with a three-day history of fever, cough and right-sided pleuritic chest pain. He smoked 20 cigarettes a day and had finished a course of tetracycline for an acute exacerbation of chronic bronchitis one week earlier. He was dyspnoeic with a temperature of 38.2°C, respiratory rate 38, pulse 138 and blood pressure of 140/80. There was clinical and radiological evidence of right upper lobe pneumonia (**1**). Blood gases on air showed pO_2 of 7.5 kPa (56 mmHg) and pCO_2 of 6.5 kPa (49 mmHg). Blood and sputum cultures were taken (**2, 3**) and the patient was started on ampicillin 1 g 6 hourly. He was successfully resuscitated from a cardiac arrest six hours later and was transferred to ITU where he was intubated and given inotrope support. He was started on intravenous erythromycin 1 g 6 hourly and the ampicillin was changed to co-amoxyclav 1.2 g 8 hourly.

Haematology:	Hb 15.4 g/dl
	WBC $22.5 \times 10^9/l$
	Neutrophils 92% with toxic granulation
Biochemistry:	Na 129 mmol/l
	K 3.5 mmol/l
	Urea 19.8 mmol/l
	Bilirubin 36 μmol/l
	Alk. phos. 236 u/l
	AST 172 u/l
	Albumin 31 g/l

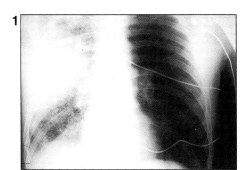

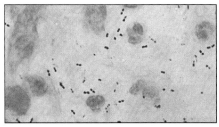

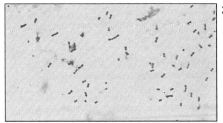

1 Chest x-ray on admission.

2 Gram stain of sputum.

3 Gram stain of blood culture at 24 hours.

Case 20

Questions

1 What does the sputum Gram stain (**2**) reveal?
2 What is the most likely identity of the organism seen in the blood culture Gram stain (**3**) and how could this be rapidly confirmed?
3 Do you agree with the initial management and would you make any changes at this stage?
4 What is the likely cause of the liver dysfunction?

Answers

1 The sputum contains numerous polymorphonuclear leucocytes, Gram positive diplococci and scanty Gram negative bacilli. The culture plates yielded a mixture of an α-haemolytic streptococcus and a lactose-fermenting coliform. These isolates were confirmed to be *Streptococcus pneumoniae* and *Escherichia coli,* respectively. *E. coli* is unlikely to cause pneumonia, but is often isolated from the upper airway of patients who have recently received antibiotics.
2 The Gram stain of the blood culture shows Gram positive diplococci which are likely to be *S. pneumoniae* in a patient with pneumonia. This could be rapidly confirmed by testing the broth supernatant with a latex agglutination test for pneumococcal antigen (**4**). This was confirmed on sub-culture, which yielded an optochin sensitive α-haemolytic mucoid growth (**5**). The mucoid appearance is due to the copious production of capsular polysaccharide which is particularly common with type III strains. Such isolates are associated with an increased mortality (30% versus 10% generally). The overall mortality from pneumococcal pneumonia has declined little in the past 40 years, despite advances in intensive care.
3 This patient had several features of severe community acquired pneumonia on admission (Box 1) and was in the category of patients that are best managed on an intensive care unit, as his subsequent progress confirmed. The initial choice of ampicillin alone was inadequate, the addition of high-dose erythromycin being prudent to cover atypical pathogens. Alternatives include the newer macrolides, such as azithromycin or clarithromycin. The change to co-amoxyclav is more questionable, but in a patient with prior chest disease *Haemophilus influenzae* is a possible pathogen which co-amoxyclav would cover more reliably than would erythromycin.

4

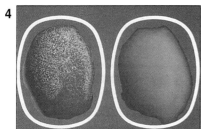

4 Latex agglutination test for pneumococcal antigen (positive on left panel).

5

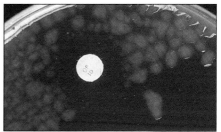

5 Sub-culture of blood showing mucoid colonies sensitive to optochin.

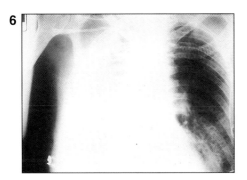

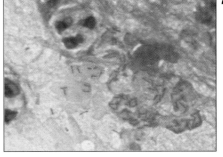

6 Chest x-ray on day 6.

7 Gram stain of tracheal aspirate on day 6.

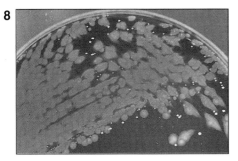

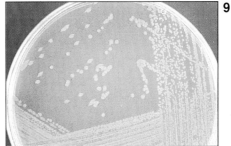

8, 9 Aerobic cultures of tracheal aspirate on blood agar (**8**) and MacConkey's medium (**9**) after 24 hours.

When the isolate is confirmed to be a penicillin sensitive *S. pneumoniae,* it is reasonable to switch to monotherapy with high dose intravenous penicillin.

4 This degree of liver dysfunction is very common in patients with severe bacterial infection of almost any type and is well documented in pneumococcal infection. The underlying cause is unclear, but it may be one manifestation of the multi-organ failure often seen in severe sepsis. It does not require further investigation at this stage, although it would be advisable to perform a clotting screen.

Progress

The patient initially responded, with reduction in fever and improvement in his blood gases. The same antibiotic regimen was continued, but his blood gases deteriorated on day 6. His most recent chest x-ray (**6**) and the microscopy and culture of a tracheal aspirate taken on day 6 are shown (**6–9**).

Questions

5 What is the likely identity of the predominant organism in the tracheal aspirate and how could this tentatively be confirmed rapidly?

6 Would you change the antimicrobial treatment at this stage, and if so how?

Case 20

Answers

5 This non-lactose fermenting organism is likely to be a *Pseudomonas* species. This can be confirmed tentatively by immediate oxidase testing (**10**). Oxidase positive organisms, such as *Ps. aeruginosa,* rapidly produce a dark purple colour when smeared onto filter paper soaked in tetramethylphenylenediamine hydrochloride. Full identification requires a detailed biochemical profile. The patient is likely to have acquired this isolate from his own flora as the relatively resistant nature of *Pseudomonas* sp. allows them to overgrow in the face of antibiotic pressure. However, the possibility of exogenous infection should also be considered. *Pseudomonas* sp. are invariably present in moist niches, such as sinks or drains, but transfer from such sites is unlikely. Humidifier traps and pools of condensation in ventilator tubing are potential sources of nosocomial transmission of Gram negative bacilli such as *Pseudomonas* sp., *Acinetobacter* sp. and *Serratia* sp. Patient-to-patient cross infection on the hands of staff is a more common route and a constant risk for the compromised patient in ITU.

6 Distinguishing between colonisation and superinfection in this context is often difficult, especially in a patient with a severe initial infection who may also have adult respiratory distress syndrome. The aspiration of increasing volumes of purulent tracheal secretions that yield a heavy growth of the suspect organism, in association with new pulmonary infiltrates and deteriorating blood gases, is highly suggestive and requires immediate treatment with an appropriate antimicrobial. However, when these findings are less clear cut, it may be preferable to withhold further antibiotics and follow developments closely; protected-brush sampling of the lower airways or bronchoalveolar lavage can be helpful in this situation. Monotherapy with quinolones, imipenem or β-lactams with high level activity against pseudomonas, such as ceftazidime or cefoperazone, is simpler and potentially less toxic than traditional treatment with a combination of an antipseudomonal penicillin and an aminoglycoside. High peak serum levels of aminoglycoside (e.g. minimum of 8 mg/l for gentamicin) are required if they are used for the treatment of pneumonia. The risk of resistance emerging on monotherapy is higher: selection of resistant mutants is not infrequent among *Pseudomonas* sp. exposed to quinolones, and constitutive resistance to a wide range of β-lactams may emerge due to stably derepressed β-lactamase production, particularly with *Enterobacter* sp.

Progress

The patient was started on intravenous ciprofloxacin 200mg bid. After initial suppression of the *Pseudomonas* sp, an isolate with an increased level of resistance emerged (**11, 12**). At this time the patient developed hypotension and oliguria, which were refractory to inotrope support, suggesting recurrent sepsis. A thorough assessment, including repeatedly negative cultures of blood and urine, changing all intravascular cannulae and a negative laparotomy, failed to reveal another focus of infection. He was started on imipenem 500 mg qid to treat the new tracheal isolate. Despite this he remained haemodynamically unstable and died 24 hours later, three weeks after admission.

Box 1: clinical and laboratory features associated with an increased risk of death in community acquired pneumonia.
British Thoracic Society, Br.J. Hosp. Med., 1993; **49,** 346–350.

If two or more of the features marked* are present, the risk of death or need for ITU management is increased 21 fold.

· **Clinical**
Respiratory rate >30/min*
Diastolic blood pressure <60 mmHg*
Age >60
Underlying disease
Confusion
Atrial fibrillation
Multilobar involvement

· **Laboratory features**
Urea >7mmol/l*
Albumin <35 g/l
pO_2 <8 kPa (60 mmHg)
Leucopenia <4.0 × 10^9/l

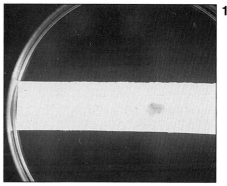

10 Positive oxidase test (see text).

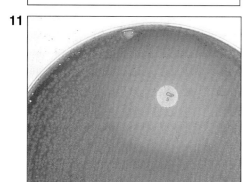

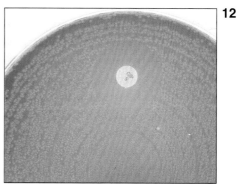

11, 12 Original (**11**) and later (**12**) isolates of pseudomonas showing reduction in zone size around a 5µg disc of ciprofloxacin.

Case 21

The febrile Indian sailor

History

A 31-year-old Indian merchant seaman is referred by the Port Health doctor with a four-day history of fever, vomiting, abdominal pain and frequent diarrhoea. He had left Delhi one month previously to join his ship in the USA before sailing, via Venezuela and Mexico, to Liverpool. His medical history includes laparotomy after a road traffic accident 10 years ago and jaundice four years ago.

On admission he looks unwell, with pulse 130, blood pressure 110/70, pyrexia spiking to 39.0°C, diffuse abdominal tenderness without peritonism, and offensive bloody diarrhoea. On re-examination the following day his pyrexia and diarrhoea persist, his liver is enlarged and tender (1) and the right lung base is dull to percussion with a pleural rub above the limit of dullness (2). Chest x-rays are shown (3, 4).

Haematology:	Hb 14.2 g/dl
	WBC 20 × 10^9/l
	Neutrophils 74% with left shift
	Platelets 229 × 10^9/l
	ESR 112 mm/hr
Biochemistry:	Na 127 mmol/l
	K 4 mmol/l
	Urea 4.8 mmol/l
	Creatinine 92 µmol/l
	Glucose 5.0 mmol/l
	Bilirubin 77 µmol/l
	AST 20 u/l
	Alk. phos. 163 u/l
	Albumin 42 g/l, total protein 76 g/l

The Port Health doctor thought the patient might have typhoid, and the initial diagnosis in hospital was infectious gastroenteritis. He was started on ampicillin intravenously.

Questions

1 What do the chest x-rays show?
2 What other diagnoses should be considered?
3 Was the initial management of his possible gastroenteritis appropriate?
4 What further investigations are essential?
5 How should he be treated?

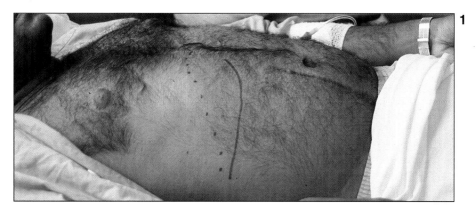

1 Tender hepatomegaly and previous laparotomy scar.

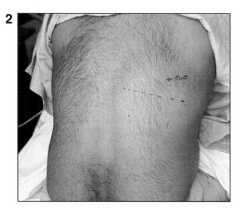

2 Dullness at right lung base (dotted line) and site of pleural rub (arrow).

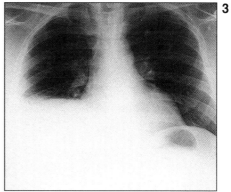

3 Chest x-ray on admission.

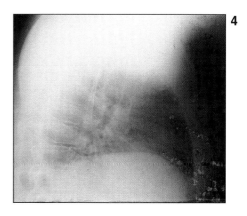

4 Right lateral chest x-ray on admission.

Case 21

Answers

1   The chest x-rays show a raised right hemidiaphragm with reactive changes in the lower right lung, suggestive of a hepatic abscess.

2   Diagnoses to consider include all causes of dysentery, especially campylobacter, shigella or amoeba, and atypical appendicitis or inflammatory bowel disease. By the next day, the history, physical signs and chest x-ray findings strongly suggest amoebic liver abscess. Bacterial liver abscess complicating appendicitis is a much less likely diagnosis.

3   Adults with bacterial or viral gastroenteritis do not usually require antibiotic treatment. Patients who are very toxic and possibly bacteraemic may merit empirical antibiotic treatment, which should cover salmonella, shigella and campylobacter, and in this case typhoid and paratyphoid. Ampicillin only covers a minority of non-typhoidal salmonellae and shigella species, and has no activity against campylobacter. The best agent for blind therapy is a quinolone, such as ciprofloxacin, with cotrimoxazole (or trimethroprim alone) as second choice to provide reasonable enteric fever cover.

4   Cultures of blood and faeces were sterile and repeated blood films for malaria were negative. Microscopy of freshly passed faeces showed numerous RBCs and WBCs, and active trophozoites of *Entamoeba histolytica* were present (**5**). The presence or absence of *E. histolytica* in faeces has little predictive value in making the diagnosis of amoebic liver abscess in a patient from an endemic area, and only a minority of patients with amoebic liver abscesses have concomitant dysentery. Ultrasound of the liver showed a hyperechoic lesion 7.5 × 8.8 cm in diameter in the upper posterior right lobe of the liver (**6**). Amoebic serology (IFAT) was weakly positive at a dilution of 1:64 (**7, 8**). Serology may be negative within two weeks of onset of symptoms in about 10% of patients and should be repeated later to confirm the diagnosis in such cases.

5   Initial empirical treatment with ampicillin was changed to metronidazole. The patient's fever and general condition improved on the third day of treatment, although right-sided pleuritic pain had become more prominent. Aspiration of the abscess was not required for diagnostic or therapeutic purposes. Aspiration is usually reserved for large abscesses, particularly for early relief of pain, but should be considered electively for the minority of abscesses that present in the left lobe of the liver, because of the risk that these will spontaneously rupture into the mediastinum or pericardium. After 5 days of metronidazole he was well enough to rejoin his ship, and was given a two-week course of diloxanide furoate to kill vegetative amoebae in the bowel (not affected by metronidazole).

This patient was not available for further follow-up, but it is likely that serial ultrasound examination of his liver would have shown persistence of the abscess cavity for several months.

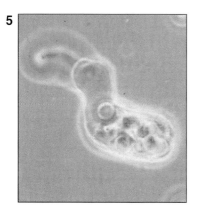

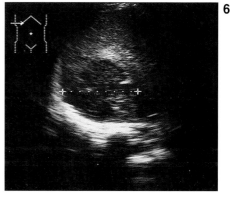

5 High power view of active trophozoite of Entamoeba histolytica with ingested red cells.

6 Ultrasound of liver showing large abscess.

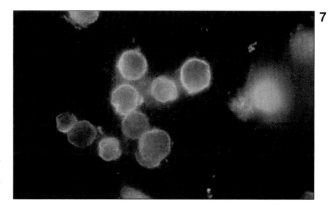

7 Positive amoebic IFAT using fixed E. histolytica trophozoites.

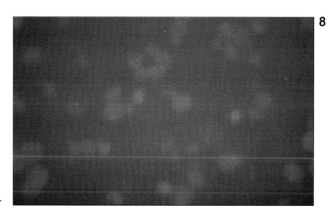

8 Negative control IFAT.

Hazardous hobbies

History

A 37-year-old man, whose hobbies include rose growing and keeping tropical fish, attends the clinic with a 10-week history of slowly progressive, non-tender, firm nodules on the right arm, starting with swelling on his right 4th finger (**1**, **2**). He has remained systemically well throughout this period.

Question

What diagnoses and investigations would you consider?

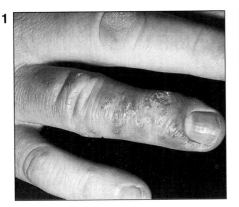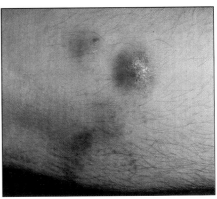

1, 2   Lesions on the patient's hand and antecubital fossa.

Answer

The physical findings are those of a chronic infection following inoculation into the finger, with nodular lymphangitis spreading up the arm. The main differential diagnosis is between infection with *Sporothrix schenckii*, a dimorphic fungus found in soil (sporotrichosis) and *Mycobacterium marinum*, an atypical mycobacterium found in swimming pools and fish tanks. Rarely, similar lesions are seen with *M. kansasii* and *Nocardia brasiliensis*.

In the absence of any discharge from the lesions which can be cultured, biopsy is essential for diagnosis. Histology (including Grocott's and Ziehl–Neelsen stains) is required – as well as culture on Sabouraud's agar and Lowenstein–Jensen media, which should be incubated for at least 8 weeks at 30°C to grow *M. marinum*.

Histology revealed non-caseating granulomata and culture yielded *M. marinum*. The patient responded to a 6-week course of cotrimoxazole. Tetracyclines could also have been used.

Headache after transplantation

History

A 47-year-old man is admitted with a history of malaise for 4 days followed by vomiting and frontal headache over the previous 36 hours. He had a cadaveric renal transplant 6 weeks previously which continues to function well with a daily regimen of cyclosporin 600 mg and prednisolone 40 mg.

Examination reveals a temperature of 39.5°C, pulse of 100 and blood pressure 100/60. There is mild neck stiffness and upper limb ataxia. He is given ceftazidime 1g 8 hourly but 12 hours later has a brief focal seizure. On re-examination he is still febrile and has generalised hypertonia and definite neck stiffness, but remains oriented with no focal neurological signs except a left VIth nerve palsy and more prominent ataxia. A rash is noted (1).

Haematology:	Hb 11.3 g/dl
	WBC 14.5 × 10⁹/l
	Neutrophils 72%, lymphocytes 12%, monocytes 10%
Biochemistry:	Na 139 mmol/l, K 2.9 mmol/l
	Urea 9.9 mmol/l, Creatinine 154 μmol/l
	Glucose 6.5 mmol/l
CSF:	RBC 30 × 10⁶/l, WBC 1050 × 10⁶/l
	Protein 1.4 g/l, Glucose 1.2 mmol/l
	Gram stain: see below (2)

Questions

1 What is the significance of the rash?
2 What are the most likely causes of the CSF findings?
3 What anti-infective treatment would be appropriate at this stage?
4 What public health measures should be considered?

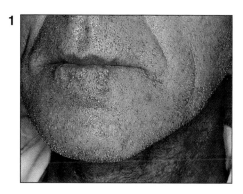

1 Rash on admission.

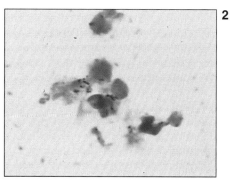

2 Gram stain of CSF.

Case 23

Answers

1 There is a vesicular rash round the mouth and on the neck typical of recurrent herpes simplex. The viral diagnosis can be confirmed by electron microscopy and culture of vesicle fluid. These infections disseminate readily in immunosuppressed patients and are an important cause of mucositis in transplant patients. However, the presence of fresh herpes simplex lesions has no correlation with central nervous system (CNS) invasion and has no positive or negative predictive value for diagnosing herpes encephalitis.

2 The Gram stain shows a predominance of polymorphonuclear cells and scanty Gram-positive bacilli which are most likely to be *Listeria monocytogenes.* Had the organisms not been seen, the common causes of bacterial meningitis, *Neisseria menigitidis, Streptococcus pneumoniae* and *Haemophilus influenzae,* should have been considered. The marked polymorphonuclear pleocytosis would be unusual in tuberculous or cryptococcal meningitis, as would the short history, although the VIth nerve palsy is suggestive of a basal meningitis. A viral meningitis can occasionally give a polymorph response of this degree, although it is uncommon and rapidly progresses to a lymphocytosis. The ataxia and VIth nerve palsy are suggestive of a brain stem encephalitis, which is a classic feature of listerial infection of the CNS. Herpes simplex encephalitis is unlikely with this degree of pleocytosis and tends to cause temporal lobe symptoms, although the manifestations are protean.

The diagnosis of listerosis was confirmed by culture of CSF and blood, yielding Gram-positive bacilli that showed a characteristic 'tumbling' motility in a hanging-drop preparation. Incubation of the isolate on an aesculin slope is a useful rapid test to differentiate *Listeria* sp. from diphtheroids, which have a similar appearance on Gram stain but are usually aesculin-negative (**3**). Some *Listeria* sp. are haemolytic (**4**), and this is used in the CAMP test which is valuable for speciation. In the CAMP test, haemolysis caused by *L. monocytogenes* (but not other species) is enhanced in the presence of a β-toxin producing strain of *Staphylococcus aureus.*

3 Antimicrobial agents with good activity against *Listeria* sp. must be started in high dose immediately. Cephalosporins are not effective – ampicillin and gentamicin are generally regarded as the agents of choice, although the utility of gentamicin in CNS infection is limited by its poor penetration of the blood–brain barrier and dose-limiting toxicity. Gentamicin may be given intrathecally but levels in brain tissue remain low. Although *Listeria* sp. are highly tolerant of ampicillin alone, there are no controlled data to support the common statement that monotherapy is likely to result in the relapse of CNS infections. Co-trimoxazole is a suitable alternative in view of its good CNS penetration.

4 The source of the listeria must be considered. In many sporadic cases it cannot be identified but it is well recognised that certain foods can become heavily colonised with listeria, which grows slowly at temperatures of +4°C and above. Refrigerated foods, especially pâté and soft cheeses (**5**), have been associated with outbreaks and 'cook-chill' foods that have been inadequately cooked or reheated have also been implicated. The public health authorities

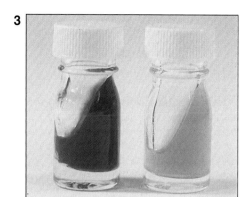

3 Positive aesculin test to distinguish Listeria sp. (dark slope on left) from most diphtheroids.

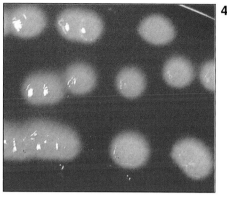

4 Haemolysis around colonies of L. monocytogenes on blood agar.

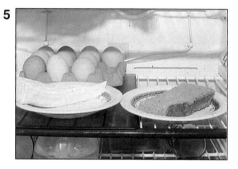

5 Possible sources of infection (for once the eggs are innocent bystanders).

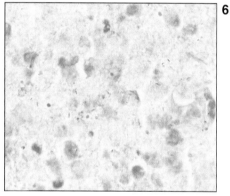

6 Brain abscess containing scanty Gram-positive bacilli (Gram stain).

should be notified as soon as cultures are provisionally identified. Person-to-person spread has been documented rarely and the patient should be nursed with enteric precautions, especially if on a ward with many immunocompromised patients.

Progress

He was given ampicillin and gentamicin but developed acute hydrocephalus due to multiple abscesses which occluded the aqueduct. His condition continued to deteriorate, despite insertion of a shunt and change of therapy to high-dose cotrimoxazole. Postmortem histology is shown above (**6**).

Case 24

Line fever

History

A 37-year-old man with a history of extensive small bowel resection for Crohn's disease presents with a 7-day history of low fever and malaise. He is receiving long-term total parenteral nutrition (TPN), which he infuses overnight at home via a Hickman catheter. On examination 2 days earlier no abnormalities had been found except for a temperature of 38.2°C. Blood for haematology, biochemical profile and culture had been collected from a peripheral vein. A swab had been taken from the catheter insertion site, which does not appear to be inflamed. Oral flucloxacillin 500 mg 8 hourly was started and he was asked to report back in 48 hours to be reviewed following receipt of the results of these investigations. On further examination, apart from a continued fever, no abnormalities are found.

Haematology: Hb 13.4 g/dl
                   WBC 12.2 × 10^9/l
                   Neutrophils 75%, lymphocytes 15%

Biochemistry: Na 137 mmol/l
                   K 4.6 mmol/l
                   Urea 4.7 mmol/l
                   Albumin 35 g/l, total protein 75 g/l
                   Alk. phos. 43 u/l
                   AST 22 u/l

Microbiology: Culture of swab from the catheter exit site grew scanty
                   coagulase negative staphylococci and diphtheroids. Blood
                   culture isolates are shown opposite (**1–3**).

Questions

1 What do the blood cultures show?
2 What is the likely source of the fever?
3 What further investigations should be undertaken?
4 How might these investigations influence your management?

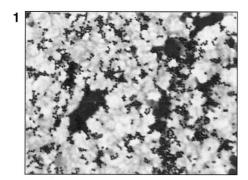

1 Gram strain of blood culture broth after incubation for 24 hours.

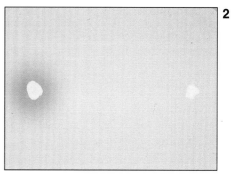

2 DNase test agar after developing with HCl. Positive control of S. aureus on left, blood culture isolate on right.

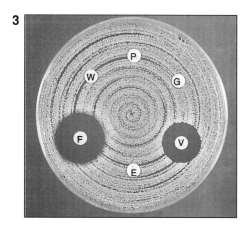

3 Disc diffusion antimicrobial sensitivity test on blood culture isolate. Disc abbreviations, clockwise: P = penicillin, G = gentamicin, V = vancomycin, E = erythromycin, F = fusidic acid, W = trimethoprim.

Answers

1 and 2   The Gram stain of the blood culture (**1**) shows Gram positive cocci in clusters, suggestive of staphylococci. *Staphylococcus aureus* is characteristically distinguished from other staphylococci by the coagulase test. Testing for DNase is an alternative method that gives similar results, and the isolate from this patient shows no surrounding halo compared to the positive control (**2**). Coagulase (DNase) negative staphylococci are found in normal skin flora and are generally of low virulence. The sensitivity plate shows that fusidic acid and vancomycin are the only active agents tested, so far. Multiple resistance to this degree is common among coagulase negative staphylococci, which are the most frequent cause of both long-term central venous catheter infection and of blood culture contamination.

The lack of inflammation or unusual bacterial flora at the catheter skin exit site does not exclude catheter-related infection. While some infections originate at the exit site, many are due to intraluminal contamination

Case 24

4 Example of pour plates, showing numerous colonies in central venous blood (left) and scanty growth in peripheral blood (right).

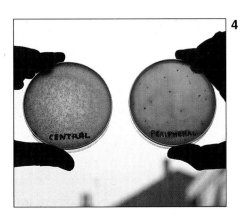

following manipulation of the junctions in the TPN administration system. Although the microbiological evidence is not conclusive at present, catheter-related infection is the most likely cause of fever in this case in the absence of any evidence of active Crohn's disease.

3   Further tests to clarify the relevance of the bacteraemia are essential. Repeat blood cultures from both the central venous catheter and a peripheral vein are helpful since the inoculum in the central venous blood will usually be higher if the catheter is the source of the bacteraemia. This can be demonstrated quantitatively by preparing pour plates (**4**). The ability to make this distinction is especially useful when the infecting organism is not a typical catheter pathogen (such as a Gram-negative organism) and the possibility of an alternative source of bacteraemia is high.

4   If repeat cultures confirm a catheter-related infection, the options are line removal or a trial of antibiotic treatment with the line *in situ*. This decision will be influenced in part by the technical difficulties envisaged in placing a new catheter and by how critical continued venous access is for the patient's management. When continued access is essential a trial of antibiotics is reasonable if both the following criteria are met:

- the infection is with an organism of low pathogenic potential, usually coagulase negative staphylococci or diphtheroids;
- there is minimal or no clinical infection at the exit site.

Infection that has extended into the skin tunnel (**5**) may be partially controlled by antimicrobials but cure is rarely achieved. Catheter infection with *S. aureus*, coliforms or yeasts usually necessitates immediate line removal as the risk of metastatic infection is high.

The antibiotic of choice in this case is vancomycin (or teicoplanin). Despite the sensitivity results, fusidic acid should not be used alone as resistance often emerges during treatment. The antibiotic must be given through the infected line and, if it is a multi-channel catheter, down each port in turn.

The full microbiological investigation of a line removed for suspected infection requires semi-quantitative sampling of both the internal and external surfaces (**6–9**). The recovery of 15 or more colonies suggests true infection rather than skin contaminants acquired during line removal.

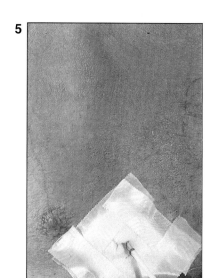

5 Severe subcutaneous tunnel infection in another patient with a Hickman catheter. Antibiotic treatment had controlled the spreading cellulitis, which had retreated from the limits shown with marker pen, but had failed to control the tunnel infection.

6–9 Microbiological processing of an infected Udall haemodialysis catheter. Intraluminal sampling by flushing with broth and surface plating (**6**). External sampling by rolling across agar plate (**7**). Tip of dialysis catheter with perforations (**8**). Result showing intraluminal colonisation (**9**). Top row: external roll cultures, positive only where perforations are present at distal third. Bottom row: intraluminal cultures, all showing heavy growth. Far right: skin insertion site, no growth.

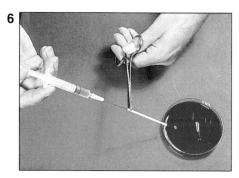

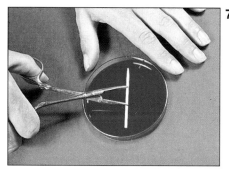

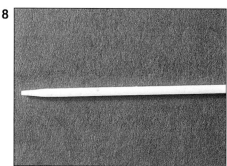

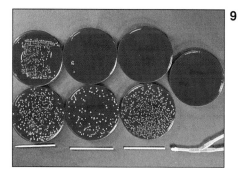

Case 25

Shock and rash

History

A 53-year-old man is referred urgently to hospital by his general practitioner after developing a petechial rash and confusion. He has been ill for 12 hours, with fever, diffuse myalgia and headache. Apart from long-standing hypertension and operations following a road traffic accident 6 years ago, he has no significant past medical history. He has not travelled abroad and none of his family or close contacts has been unwell recently.

Examination reveals an ill man with a temperature of 39.8°C, pulse of 138, blood pressure 90/50, and a respiratory rate of 26. He has an obvious rash which is most prominent on the face (**1**) and feet (**2**), with smaller petechial lesions on the trunk. Diffuse crepitations are heard in both lung fields and his heart sounds are normal. Abdominal examination is normal apart from a midline laparotomy scar. He is drowsy but able to respond to commands and he has no neck stiffness or focal neurological signs. His limb muscles are tender but there is no bone or joint tenderness.

Haematology:	Hb 12.4 g/dl
	WBC 16.7 × 10⁹/l
	Neutrophils 92%, lymphocytes 6%
	Platelets 460 × 10⁹/l
	Blood film: shown opposite (**3**, **4**)
Biochemistry:	Na 135 mmol/l
	K 4.5 mmol/l
	Urea 8.4 mmol/l
	Creatinine 135 μmol/l
	Bilirubin 25 μmol/l
	AST 140 u/l
	Alk. phos. 137 u/l
Blood gases: (room air)	pH 7.31, Base excess -17 mmol/l, pO$_2$ 9.9 kPa (74 mmHg), pCO$_2$ 5.7 kPa (43 mmHg)
Radiology:	Chest x-ray shown opposite (**5**)

Questions

1 What are the possible causes of his skin rash?
2 What abnormalities are present in the blood films?
3 What is the relevance of his medical past history?
4 What treatment would you institute?

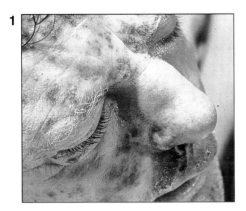
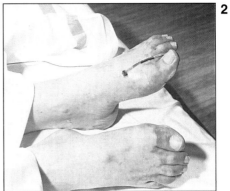

1, 2 Rash shortly after arrival at hospital.

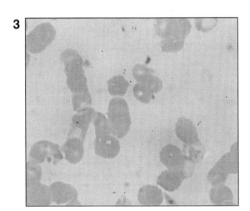
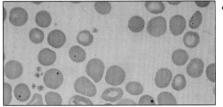

3, 4 Selected fields of peripheral blood film on admission.

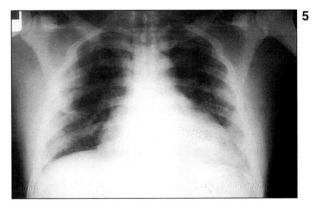

5 Chest x-ray on admission.

Case 25

Answers

1   The classical cause of a rapidly progressive purpuric skin rash is infection with *Neisseria meningitidis*. Severe infections with other organisms, especially *Streptococcus pneumoniae* and *Haemophilus influenzae*, can occasionally give a similar appearance. Vasculitis of non-infective origin rarely develops so rapidly. The chest x-ray shows cardiomegaly and diffuse pulmonary infiltrates compatible with pulmonary infection or early adult respiratory distress syndrome. There were no signs of endocarditis but CSF obtained 24 hours after admission showed changes of treated pyogenic meningitis.

2   The blood film (**4**) shows small blue inclusions in red cells. These are Howell–Jolly bodies, which are found in patients with hyposplenism. The other film (**3**) reveals blue-staining diplococci in the background, the morphology of which is strongly suggestive of *S. pneumoniae*. Organisms are only directly visible in blood films of patients with very high-grade bacteraemias, which are most often found in asplenic subjects. Phagocytosed organisms are more readily seen in buffy coat preparations.

3   He had a splenectomy following his road traffic accident. The clues to this are the haematological changes, including the high platelet count in the presence of presumed sepsis.

4.   The diagnosis of pneumococcal septicaemia in an asplenic patient was confirmed by isolation of pneumococci from blood cultures taken prior to administration of intravenous benzyl penicillin 1.8 g 6 hourly. In countries where penicillin-resistant pneumococci are prevalent, cefotaxime 2 g 8 hourly or vancomycin 1 g 12 hourly would be appropriate choices for therapy of suspected severe *S. pneumoniae* infection.

Asplenic patients are at risk of overwhelming infection, especially with pneumococci. The risk is greatest in children and in the first year after splenectomy. Patients with sickle cell disease are at increased risk of severe pneumococcal infection, particularly in childhood. This is due not only to the progressive loss of splenic function in sickle cell disease but additionally to a defect in the alternative complement pathway.

The interval between the onset of vague, flu-like symptoms and death may be as little as 12 hours, and despite appropriate antibiotics and aggressive supportive care the mortality rate is very high. This risk can be reduced only by prophylactic measures. Pneumococcal vaccine should be given to all patients, preferably at least 2 weeks or more before elective splenectomy, or after recovery from surgery involving emergency splenectomy. Whenever possible, splenic tissue should be conserved after trauma. Chemoprophylaxis with penicillin is now established to reduce morbidity in children with sickle cell disease and should be considered for other asplenic patients. Early self-treatment of fever with penicillin or erythromycin is another option.

Malaria infection in asplenic patients follows a fulminant course and such patients should be discouraged from visiting malarious areas. Other infections that may be more severe in asplenic patients include those caused by *H. influenzae*, *Capnocytophaga canimorus* (DF-2) and *Babesia* sp.

Case 26

Open wide

History

A 4-year-old girl is admitted to hospital with a 48-hour history of sore throat, nasal discharge, fever and anorexia. Over the previous 24 hours she has become hoarse and has had difficulty swallowing. She has never been outside Britain. On examination she has marked halitosis, a temperature of 38.2°C and a pulse of 98. Her other physical signs are shown below (**1–3**).

Questions

1   What is the diagnosis?
2   How would you confirm this diagnosis?
3   How would you manage this patient?
4   What additional measures should be taken as soon as possible?

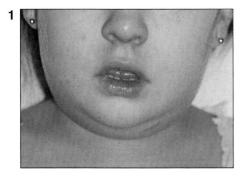
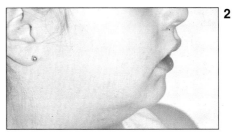

1, 2 The patient on admission. (By permission of JT Macfarlane et al)

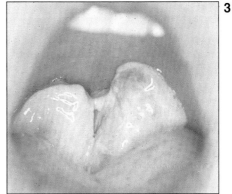

3   Throat on admission.

Case 26

Answers

1   The fauces and soft palate are covered by a thick, grey membrane – the classical presentation of diphtheria. The 'bull neck' appearance due to oedema and cervical lymphadenopathy is also typical of this condition and is a marker of severe disease. The main differential diagnosis is faucial mononucleosis due to Epstein–Barr virus infection (anginose glandular fever) in which the membrane is restricted to the tonsils and remains a creamy white, with peripheral blood usually containing atypical lymphocytes. Streptococcal pharyngitis is characteristically more intense and associated with a high fever.

2   The diagnosis is confirmed by culture of *Corynebacterium diphtheriae* from the throat and by demonstration that the isolate can produce diphtheria toxin. *C. diphtheriae* is most easily recovered on selective media containing potassium tellurite, which suppresses normal throat flora and imparts a grey-black colour to the colony (**4**). The species is subdivided into three types – *C. diphtheriae* var. *gravis*, var. *intermedius* and var. *mitis* – on the basis of colonial morphology, sugar fermentation reactions and haemolytic potential. Production of toxin by the isolate is verified using the Elek test (**5**). Diphtheria toxin kills mammalian cells by blocking protein synthesis, and is responsible for the production of the necrotic membrane.

3   There are five important aspects of management:

- Close observation of the airway, which can become obstructed by aspiration of dislodged membrane. If there is laryngeal or tracheal involvement, early intubation or tracheostomy is required.
- Antimicrobial therapy is needed to prevent further toxin production and transmission of infection to others. Benzyl penicillin or erythromycin should be given for 14 days.
- Neutralisation of free toxin with diphtheria antitoxin. While the damage due to intracellular toxin cannot be reversed, further uptake can be blocked and antitoxin should be given as soon as possible. The antiserum is raised in horses and there is a significant risk of hypersensitivity reactions, including serum sickness, which preclude its use for prophylaxis of contacts. A small test dose should first be given intradermally or applied to the conjunctiva.
- Observation for late complications due to systemic toxin. These are principally cardiotoxicity (arrhythmias and heart failure due to myocarditis) and neurotoxicity (paralysis of the soft palate, or polyneuritis). Either may develop as long as three months after the acute illness.
- The patient should be managed with bed rest in respiratory isolation. Staff should wear gowns, gloves and masks and the room should be under negative pressure.

4   A single case of diphtheria necessitates screening of all household and school or nursery contacts to detect secondary carriers and any index case. Throat swabs should be collected from contacts and erythromycin should be given for 7 days to those with positive cultures. Further swabs should be taken

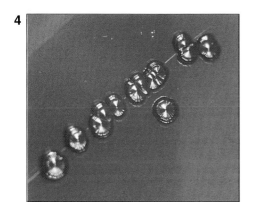

4 Corynebacterium diphtheriae var. gravis colonies on potassium tellurite agar, showing typical 'daisy-head' appearance.

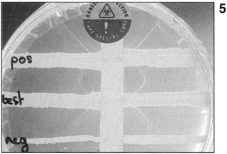

5 Elek test. Antitoxin diffusing out from vertical strip of paper forms complexes with toxin produced by horizontal streaks of positive control organism and of test organism, to produce visible precipitation arcs.

2 weeks after completion of antibiotics to ensure eradication.

The immunisation history of contacts should be checked and any who have not been immunised should be given a primary course (3 doses); they should also receive erythromycin before results of their throat swabs are available. Immunised contacts should be given a single booster dose of diphtheria vaccine. For both primary immunisation and booster doses, standard-strength vaccine should be used only for children under the age of 10. Contacts over this age are likely to experience vaccine reactions from standard-strength vaccine if they have pre-existing immunity, and so should be given low-dose (adult) vaccine. The risk of reactions to the low-dose vaccine is low enough for it to be given without prior tests for immunity – Schick intradermal tests or measurement of serum neutralising antibodies are often difficult to arrange quickly in this situation.

Progress

In view of the severity of her illness with a 'bull neck', the girl was given a high dose (80,000 units) of diphtheria antitoxin and was put on a course of intravenous benzyl penicillin. She made an uneventful recovery over the next 2 weeks with no late cardiac or neural toxicity. Screening the playgroup she attended revealed the index case, who had returned from West Africa 6 weeks earlier. Diphtheria is rarely seen in developed countries and a high index of suspicion must be maintained in order to diagnose less severe cases. Adults planning long stays in areas with a high incidence of diphtheria are advised to have a low-strength booster dose of vaccine prior to departure.

Case 27

Wanderers

History

Two women presented with slowly moving, itchy raised skin rashes shortly after going on beach holidays in the West Indies. One patient had a solitary lesion on the foot (**1**) and the second had multiple lesions on her trunk (**2**).

Question

What is the diagnosis and how should the patients be treated?

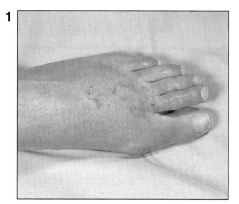 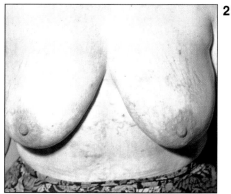

1 Itchy lesion on the foot.

2 Multiple lesions on the trunk.

Answer

Both patients had cutaneous larva migrans ('creeping eruption') due to invasion of the skin by third-stage larvae of the dog hookworm, *Ancylostoma caninum,* or the cat hookworm, *A. braziliensis.* Skin penetration occurs on parts of the body (usually the foot) that have been in direct contact with warm, moist soil or sand contaminated by animal faeces. Animal hookworms are not adapted for the human host and move slowly in the upper dermis, provoking the formation of characteristic pruritic serpiginous lesions that may be single or multiple. No investigations are needed to confirm the diagnosis.

Single lesions can be treated with topical ethyl chloride but are best managed by application of topical thiabendazole. Freezing the lesion with liquid nitrogen is less effective and can induce pain and blistering. Oral thiabendazole is moderately effective but has numerous unpleasant side-effects, including nausea, dizziness, feelings of depersonalisation and occasional frank psychosis. Oral albendazole is well-tolerated and the second patient was cured by a 3-day course of 400 mg twice daily. Single or lower doses of albendazole are probably equally effective. Limited experience suggests that a single oral dose of ivermectin may be a useful alternative.

Case 28

A young man with a cough

History

A 29-year-old homosexual man presented in 1987 with a 3-week history of progressive dyspnoea on exertion, dry cough, retrosternal pain on inspiration, fever and weight loss. An oral 'penicillin' prescribed by his general practitioner had not relieved his symptoms but had caused a mild drug rash.

Examination revealed a toxic, centrally cyanosed man who was short of breath at rest. His temperature was 39.5°C, pulse 110, blood pressure 100/70 and respiratory rate 32. Fine crackles were heard over both lung fields and a painless rash was noted on one arm (1).

Haematology:	Hb 10.5 g/dl, WBC 4.1×10^9/l Neutrophils 82%, lymphocytes 10%, monocytes 4%, Platelets 140×10^9/l
Biochemistry:	Na 130 mmol/l, K 4.1 mmol/l Urea 8.4 mmol/l, Creatinine 128 μmol/l
Blood gases: *(room air)*	pO_2 6.51 kPa (49 mmHg), pCO_2 4.2 kPa (32 mmHg)
Microbiology:	Gram stain of sputum showed polymorphs, Gram-positive cocci in clusters and Gram-negative coccobacilli

Questions

1 What is the diagnosis and significance of the skin rash (1)?
2 What is the differential diagnosis of his pneumonia (2)?
3 How would you investigate this further?
4 How should he be managed?

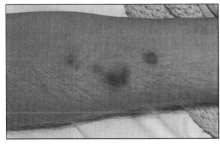

1 Painless raised lesions on forearm.

2 Chest x-ray on admission.

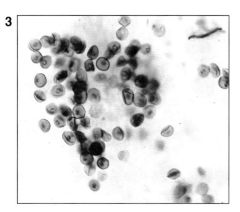 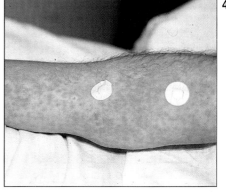

3 Typical 'cysts' of P. carinii in BAL fluid (Grocott stain, high power).

4 Itchy papular rash caused by cotrimoxazole.

Answers

1   The skin lesion is Kaposi's sarcoma and in this clinical context suggests that he has AIDS. In the absence of visceral or generalised skin involvement, chemotherapy is not usually required. This patient initially camouflaged his lesion with make-up and subsequently had local radiotherapy.

2   The chest x-ray showed bilateral shadowing, pronounced enough on the left to suggest lobar consolidation. He had a severe community-acquired pneumonia with several clinical features suggesting HIV infection. The most likely diagnosis is *Pneumocystis carinii* pneumonia (PCP). The contribution of the organisms seen in the sputum Gram stain is less certain, but bacterial causes including *Haemophilus influenzae* and *Streptococcus pneumonia* should be considered. The clinical and radiological picture is less suggestive of other pulmonary infections such as tuberculosis, CMV pneumonitis, cryptococcosis or toxoplasmosis. Any of these pathogens could be infecting lung tissue infiltrated by Kaposi's sarcoma.

3   Sputum culture yielded a heavy growth of *H. influenzae* and a scanty growth of *Staphylococcus aureus,* and blood cultures were sterile. Processing of his sputum for possible PCP gave equivocal results, and bronchoscopy was undertaken when his condition had stabilised three days after admission. Typical *P. carinii* was seen in bronchoalveolar lavage (BAL) fluid (**3**) and transbronchial biopsy specimens, prolonged culture of which did not yield mycobacteria or fungi. This patient presented at a time when local experience with sputum induction was limited. The induction of distal airways secretions with nebulised hypertonic saline has now replaced bronchoalveolar lavage in the initial investigation of patients with suspected PCP. The sensitivity and specificity of microscopy of the expectorated secretions have been improved by the availability of monoclonal antibody-based immunofluorescent stains. PCR techniques are promising but are not yet widely available. Serological tests are of no value in individual patient diagnosis.

4   He was given 35% oxygen which improved his pO$_2$ to 9.6 kPa (72 mmHg) and he was treated with high-dose intravenous cotrimoxazole to cover PCP and bacterial pneumonia. Intravenous hydrocortisone, followed by a short course of oral prednisolone, was also given because he had several indicators of severe PCP, including hypoxia <8 kPa (60 mmHg) not rising above 10 kPa on 35% oxygen, tachypnoea >30, and possible coexistent bacterial infection. He responded well but developed an itchy rash on day 8 of treatment (4). This became worse, necessitating a change of therapy on day 14 to nebulised pentamidine isethionate, which was given daily until his discharge home on day 22. Clindamycin or intravenous pentamidine could have been used as alternatives.

His HIV-positive status was confirmed by several different ELISA techniques and he had high serum levels of p24 antigen. His CD4+ T-lymphocyte count was 55 × 10^6/l, with a CD4:CD8 ratio of 0.12 (normal 1–3). He was given zidovudine 200 mg 8 hourly, and secondary prophylaxis against PCP was prescribed in the form of nebulised pentamidine 300 mg every 2–3 weeks, as he was intolerant of a low-dose oral cotrimoxazole challenge. Prophylaxis against PCP should be offered to all HIV-positive individuals with a CD4 count <200 ×10^6/l or who have symptoms of late-stage HIV infection.

Over the next 14 months he was treated with fluconazole for candida oesophagitis, and with acyclovir for recurrent oral herpes simplex infections. He defaulted from follow-up but was re-admitted in a debilitated state with severe watery diarrhoea for 5 weeks, associated with weight loss of 8 kg. Faecal culture was unremarkable but Ziehl–Neelsen stains of faeces (5) and rectal biopsy (6) revealed the cause of his decline.

Questions

5   What is the cause of his diarrhoea?
6   How should it be managed?

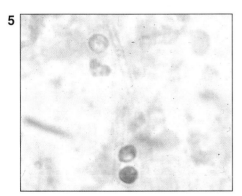

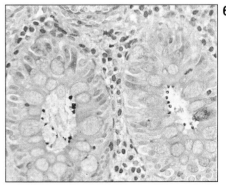

5   Ziehl–Neelsen stain of faeces (high power).

6   Rectal biopsy (PAS).

Case 28

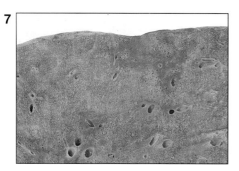

7 Lung at autopsy, showing patches of Kaposi's sarcoma.

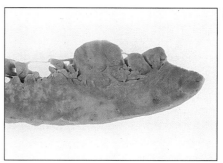

8 Heart at autopsy, showing pale areas of myocardium involved with toxoplasmosis.

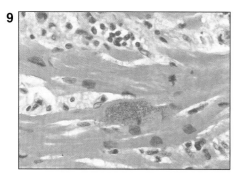

9 High-power view of myocardium containing tissue cysts of Toxoplasma gondii (haematoxylin & eosin).

Answers

5 and 6 The faecal smear shows typical oocysts of *Cryptosporidium* sp. Cryptosporidial infection is the cause of prolonged diarrhoea in about 30% of patients with late AIDS and has a gloomy prognosis. Cryptosporidiosis acquired earlier in the course of HIV infection may settle spontaneously or improve after antiretroviral treatment is begun. Supportive treatment includes rehydration and encouraging the patient to maintain an adequate calorific intake. The role of intravenous or nasogastric hyperalimentation is currently controversial. Controlled trials have so far failed to show therapeutic benefit from any antimicrobial treatment, despite initial optimism for numerous compounds.

The patient required increasing doses of long-acting morphine (and anti-emetics), which only partially relieved his diarrhoea. He developed patchy shadowing throughout both lung fields and died of presumed bronchopneumonia. At autopsy both lungs were infiltrated with Kaposi's sarcoma (**7**) and there was extensive myocardial involvement with toxoplasmosis (**8, 9**).

In retrospect, serology for toxoplasma infection had been positive at his initial presentation. We now offer chemoprophylaxis to patients with positive toxoplasma serology and low CD4 counts. If they are not already taking cotrimoxazole or Fansidar® for PCP prophylaxis, or cannot tolerate sulphur compounds, clindamycin (with pyrimethamine if tolerated) can be used.

A Cambodian with a neck-swelling

History

A 23-year-old woman of Cambodian origin presents with a non-tender neck-swelling, which has enlarged over 1 month. Apart from a vague history of fever there are no systemic symptoms. A chest x-ray on arrival in the UK 6 months earlier had been passed as normal and she does not admit to any significant past medical problems.

Examination reveals a healthy young woman with a fluctuant mobile swelling on one side of the neck (**1**). She has no other lymphadenopathy and examination of her teeth, pharynx, liver and spleen is normal.

Haematology: Hb 11.1 g/dl
WBC 5.6 x 10⁹
Neutrophils 46%, lymphocytes 35%, eosinophils 17%
Platelets 400 × 10⁹/l

Liver function: Bilirubin 18 μmol/l, AST 50 u/l, Alk. phos. 173 u/l

Chest x-ray: Normal

Tuberculin test: Illustrated (**2**)

She is given anti-tuberculous therapy and 6 weeks later has a brief generalised convulsion. Following this she has no focal neurological signs.

Questions

1 Which features do not fit with a diagnosis of tuberculosis?
2 Should the neck lesion be biopsied?
3 What anti-tuberculous medication would you prescribe and for how long?
4 What precautions should be taken before prescribing?
5 Why did she have a convulsion?

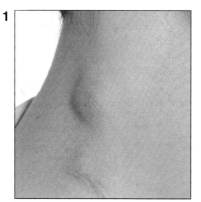

1   Neck of patient.

2   View of arm 72 hours after intradermal injection of 1 unit of tuberculin.

Case 29

Answers

1 The presentation is typical of tuberculous lymphadenopathy, which involves a single node in about 50% of cases, with a normal chest x-ray in 90%. The scar below the swelling suggests previous treatment for the same problem. The differential diagnosis includes actinomycosis, cat scratch disease, lymphoma and metastasis, all of which are extremely unlikely in this patient. The only atypical feature is the eosinophilia, which suggests atopy or helminth infection. Gnathostomiasis usually presents with more transient swellings near or on the face or on limbs and is unlikely. Examination of her faeces revealed ova of *Ascaris lumbricoides* (**3**) and *Trichuris trichuria* (**4**) which responded to treatment with mebendazole.

2 Although the strongly positive tuberculin test supports the diagnosis, diagnostic aspiration or biopsy for culture is essential to confirm the diagnosis and identify the species and drug sensitivity of the mycobacterium. The risk of local sinus formation after incision is negligible with modern chemotherapy. There is a 10–20% chance that *Mycobacterium tuberculosis* isolated from a patient from this area will be resistant to at least one first-line drug, especially if chemotherapy has been given in the past. Biopsy and culture are particularly important in HIV-positive patients, when the differential diagnosis includes lymphomas and Kaposi's sarcoma, and non-tuberculous mycobacteria are more likely to be involved. The lymph node biopsy (**5**) showed caseation and giant cells but no acid-fast bacilli. Culture of the biopsy material yielded *M. tuberculosis* resistant to streptomycin but sensitive to other first-line drugs.

3 Treatment should consist of at least 3 drugs in the initial phase followed by at least 2 drugs for several months. She was given the regimen currently recommended in Britain: that is, 2 months of rifampicin, isoniazid and pyrazinamide, followed by 4 months of rifampicin and isoniazid, which should result in >95% cure. In view of the possibility of drug resistance, it might have been more appropriate to have given a more intensive 4-drug regimen such as rifampicin, isoniazid, pyrazinamide and ethambutol for the first 2 months.

4 Her hepatic and renal function were already known to be normal. She was warned that rifampicin would make her urine and tears turn orange and could also render her oral contraception ineffective. She was asked to report any paraesthesia (isoniazid) or joint pains, as pyrazinamide-induced gout is more common in people of Asian origin. If she had been prescribed ethambutol, her colour vision and visual fields should have been checked before and during treatment and she should have been asked to report any visual problem. A pregnancy test was negative and she had an IUCD inserted. Pregnancy would not be a contraindication for the drugs that she received, but use of streptomycin should be avoided.

5 Her fits were due to an intracranial tuberculoma (**6**). Reactive swelling of infected nodes and tuberculomata is common during the initial phase of treatment and a small proportion (<5%) of patients develop fits for this reason, typically in the 2nd month of treatment. The chemotherapy should be continued, subject to the drug sensitivity profile which is usually available by 6 weeks, and anticonvulsant therapy may be indicated. The interaction

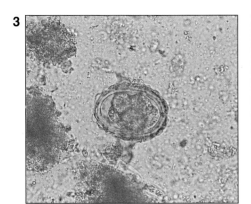

3 Ovum of Ascaris lumbricoides in unstained wet preparation of faeces (size 40 × 60 μm).

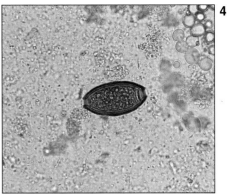

4 Trichuris trichuria ovum in unstained wet preparation of faeces (size 20 × 50 μm).

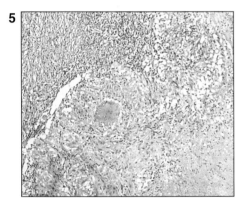

5 Histology of lymph node biopsy (haematoxylin & eosin), showing edge of necrotic area in lower right corner with adjacent giant cell.

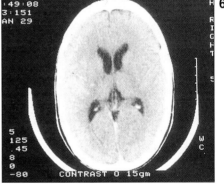

6 CT scan of patient after convulsion, showing small tuberculomata with surrounding oedema.

between the intrahepatic metabolism of phenytoin and rifampicin is unpredictable and patients taking phenytoin should be monitored closely for toxicity. The role of steroids is not clear, but a short course of dexamethasone may be indicated for an enlarging tuberculoma, especially if fits recur.

Case 30

Exotica

History

Two British soldiers presented with skin lesions after a 6-month tour of duty in Belize. The first soldier developed a solitary painless ulcer on his wrist (**1**). The second patient had several nodular lesions on his hand and wrist which had gradually enlarged (**2**). Both were otherwise in excellent health.

Questions

1 What is the infecting organism and how would you confirm this?
2 What management is appropriate?

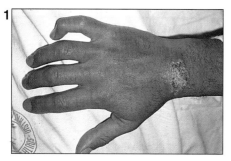

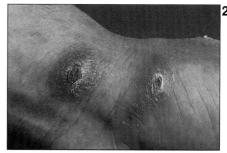

1 Solitary lesion on wrist.

2 Multiple lesions.

Answers

1 The diagnosis is cutaneous leishmaniasis, caused in this area by *Leishmania braziliensis*, *L. mexicana* or *L. amazonensis*, transmitted by the bite of sandflies (*Lutzomyia* sp.). The differential diagnosis includes tuberculosis, leprosy and blastomycoses, but these are unlikely in these patients. The diagnosis in the first case was confirmed by visualization of leishmania amastigotes within macrophages in material aspirated from the edge of the lesion. Subsequent culture of this material on NNN (Novy–MacNeal–Nicolle) medium yielded promastigotes which could not be speciated. Aspiration and culture of the lesions of the second patient were unsuccessful, but biopsy showed a granulomatous reaction and a few leishmania amastigotes. The second patient had a positive leishmanin skin test, supporting the diagnosis. Serological tests (IFAT) were negative in both cases.
2 Cutaneous leishmaniasis acquired in the Mediterranean littoral, Africa, the Middle East or the Indian subcontinent does not usually disseminate or require specific chemotherapy. However, *L. braziliensis* can cause progressive mucocutaneous destruction. Both these patients received a successful three week course of intravenous sodium stibogluconate because *L. braziliensis* could not be ruled out as the infecting species.

A dyspnoeic drug user

History

A 27-year-old man was admitted to hospital with a 3-week history of progressive dyspnoea on exertion, cough productive of dirty sputum and poorly defined chest pain. He took 60 ml of methadone syrup every day, and supplemented this with regular intravenous injections of amphetamine and occasional intravenous injections of resuspended temazepam capsules or heroin. He smoked 20 cigarettes a day but did not drink alcohol. Despite injecting for 5 years, his only previous hospitalisation was for drainage of an injection abscess in the groin 2 years previously. He denied sharing needles and did not have a regular sexual partner.

Examination revealed a pale, ill man with poor dentition. His temperature was 39°C, pulse 100, blood pressure 100/70, and respiratory rate 18. There were obvious v waves in the jugular venous pulse but no cardiac murmurs were audible over the widespread coarse crackles throughout both lung fields. There was moderate lymphadenopathy in both axillae and groins but recent injection sites in both groins were clean and non-tender. All pulses were present, there was no rash, and fundoscopy was normal.

Haematology:	Hb 7.1 g/dl
	WBC $7.4 \times 10^9/l$
	Neutrophils 92%
	Platelets $100 \times 10^9/l$
	ESR 102 mm/hr
Biochemistry:	Na 127 mmol/l
	K 3.2 mmol/l
	Urea 8.2 mmol/l
	Albumin 30 g/l

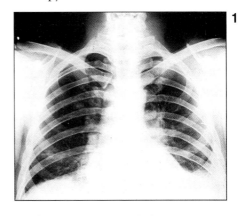

1   Chest x-ray on admission.

Questions

1 What abnormalities are visible on the chest x-ray (**1**)?
2 What is the diagnosis?
3 What organisms would you expect to find in blood cultures and what antibiotic therapy would you prescribe?
4 What other investigations and treatment would you institute on admission?
5 What is the likely prognosis?

Case 31

Answers

1   The chest x-ray shows consolidation and/or effusion in the left base, and multiple rounded opacities in both lung fields. The opacity in the right lung base contains a possible air fluid level, suggestive of abscess (**2**).

2   The diagnosis is right-sided endocarditis with multiple septic emboli to both lungs and significant tricuspid valve damage. The presentation of this patient is typical, and the tricuspid valve is the seat of infection in over 90% of such cases.

3   There are many potential sources of infection, depending on the drug-injecting technique of the user. Primary contamination of the drug mixture, including the substances used to 'cut' the pure compound, is rare and most infections are due to the use of non-sterile diluents, filtering through non-sterile cotton or cigarette filters, re-use of old syringes and needles, and the introduction of organisms associated with superficial or deep infections at the injection site. This patient had obvious dental sepsis which may be the source of infection; the common practice of licking the needle before injecting also introduces mouth organisms, particularly *Streptococcus milleri*. The use of lemon juice as a diluent carries a specific risk of introducing *Candida* sp., typically species other than *C. albicans*. Right-sided endocarditis in injecting drug users may be polymicrobial with over 10 concurrent infecting organisms reported in rare cases. *Staphylococcus aureus* is present in over 70% of cases, with other Gram-positive cocci in over 10%. Associated Gram-negative organisms include *Pseudomonas* sp., which should also be covered by initial empirical therapy in geographical areas where this is common.

The patient was given high doses of intravenous penicillin and flucloxacillin with low-dose gentamicin to cover the bacteria mentioned, pending results of blood cultures. Vancomycin would have been an alternative for the β-lactams if there had been any evidence to suggest that multiply resistant staphylococci were likely to be involved or if the patient had been allergic to penicillin. There were no specific clinical signs to suggest the need for empirical antifungal therapy.

4 and 5   Six sets of blood cultures were taken and an echocardiogram confirmed the presence of a large vegetation on the tricuspid valve (**3**). There was no evidence of left-sided disease, which has important prognostic significance. Thirty-six hours later, *S. aureus, S. milleri* and *S. pneumoniae* were isolated from blood cultures. The man's fever decreased but had not returned to normal by the seventh hospital day, when there was radiological evidence of further emboli to the lungs followed by a spontaneous pyopneumothorax, which was drained with a wide-bore tube (**4**). At this point, *Bacteroides* (*Prevotella*) *melaninogenicus,* resistant to penicillin, was isolated from the anaerobic sub-culture of the admission blood cultures plated on kanamycin blood agar, and metronidazole was added to the regimen. *S. milleri* was present in the blood cultures up to the 14th day and *S. aureus* continued to be isolated from blood cultures until the 21st day, when drug fever supervened and his therapy was changed to vancomycin, fusidic acid and metronidazole. He developed right-sided heart failure and further septic emboli but was refused surgery on the grounds that his heart failure was too severe to survive bypass.

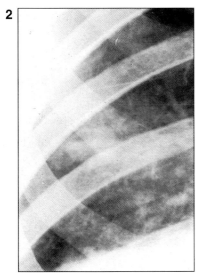

2 Chest x-ray on admission.

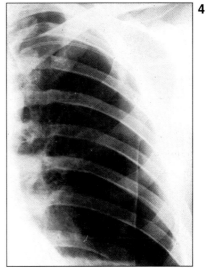

4 Spontaneous left pyopneumothorax on day 7 of admission.

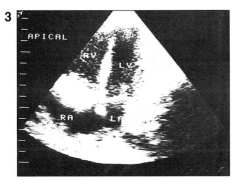

3 Transthoracic echocardiogram on
day after admission.

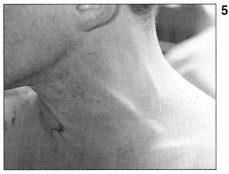

5 The patient 5 years later, with full
neck veins while sitting upright.

The indications for surgery for right-sided endocarditis in drug users are much less clear than for left-sided endocarditis. This patient had three relative indications: worsening heart failure, continued septic emboli, and persistent *S. aureus* bacteraemia – despite adequate therapy (confirmed by MICs and high bactericidal titres in his serum). Right-sided endocarditis has a low overall mortality rate of about 10% compared to over 50% for staphylococcal left-sided endocarditis. This patient left hospital after a total of 82 days. Five years later he was still abusing drugs and has cardiac cirrhosis associated with severe tricuspid incompetence (5).

Spot diagnosis 2

Case A

A 40-year-old man was admitted to hospital with a 4-day history of fever, non-specific headache and myalgia. Two days prior to admission he had noticed a rash on his arms and legs which subsequently spread to his trunk but was not itchy or painful. He had no respiratory or gastrointestinal symptoms and his past history was unremarkable. He had just returned from a camping holiday in Wales, but did not recollect being bitten by any insects or ticks.

He looked unwell with a flushed face, temperature of 38.5°C, pulse of 100 and blood pressure of 130/70. He had a generalised punctate erythematous macular rash (1–3) and moderate lymphadenopathy in the neck and groins. There was no neck stiffness, conjunctivitis, oropharyngeal abnormality, synovitis or hepatosplenomegaly. Chest x-ray and serum biochemistry were normal.

Haematology: Hb 16.5 g/dl
WBC 3.5×10^9/l
Neutrophils 79%, lymphocytes 8%, monocytes 8%
Platelets 73×10^9/l
ESR 6 mm/hr

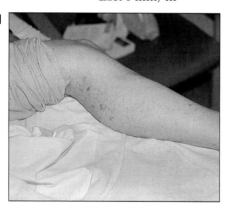

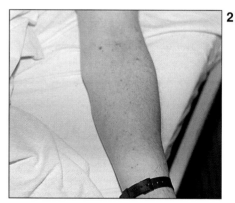

1, 2 Discrete punctate macular rash on limbs of first patient.

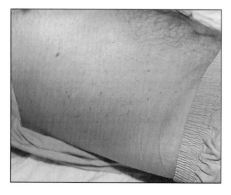

3 Trunk of first patient.

Case B

A week after the first patient was admitted a 16-year-old boy was referred by his general practitioner for diagnosis of a presumed viral illness of 6 days' duration. Initial nausea, malaise and retro-orbital headache were accompanied by the appearance of an itchy rash on his legs. The itching settled but the rash spread to his arms and trunk, sparing his hands and feet, and his mother thought his face looked flushed. He had noticed swollen glands in his groins and neck. He was prescribed oral penicillin by his general practitioner for pharyngeal erythema noted on the second day of the illness. His past history included chickenpox, rubella and measles. Further questioning revealed that he had been to the same school camp as the first patient and that several other pupils in his class had been diagnosed as having glandular fever.

He looked well and was apyrexial. A reticular rash was present on his trunk, arms and legs (4) and there was non-tender enlargement of the suboccipital, posterior cervical and inguinal lymph nodes. There were no other physical abnormalities. Results of blood tests taken by his general practitioner on the third day of illness showed normal serum biochemistry, a negative Paul Bunnel test and the following:

Haematology: Hb 14.4 g/dl
WBC 2.7×10^9/l
Neutrophils 63%, lymphocytes 22%, monocytes 10%
Platelets 216×10^9/l
ESR 4 mm/hr

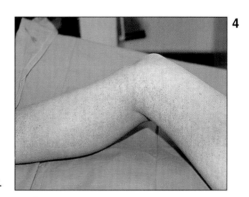

4

4   Rash on leg of second patient.

Questions

1   What is the differential diagnosis?
2   What investigations are required?
3   What other syndromes are caused by the infecting agent?
4   What advice should be given to close contacts who are pregnant?

Case 32

Answers

1, 2   Meningococcal infection must always be considered in a patient with headache, fever and a rash. Immediate lumbar puncture of the first patient was normal and initial empirical treatment with benzyl penicillin was discontinued. Cultures of CSF and blood were sterile. The history and low white count with lymphopenia are more suggestive of a viral or rickettsial illness; the degree of thrombocytopenia was not severe enough to account for the petechial appearance of his rash. The lack of prodromal respiratory illness or pronounced conjunctivitis, combined with the distribution of rash with flushed facial appearance and lymphadenopathy, is most suggestive of rubella or parvovirus B19 infection. The rash of rubella may have a papular component and typically spreads from the face to trunk, has a pinker appearance and is more confluent (**5, 6**). Neither patient had arthralgia, which may complicate either infection.

Both patients had parvovirus B19 infection, confirmed by the detection of specific IgM antibodies, negative tests for IgM antibodies to rubella and positive tests for IgG rubella antibodies. Parvoviruses are single-stranded DNA viruses 22 nm in diameter. DNA hybridisation techniques for the diagnosis of parvovirus B19 infection have been described but were not available; newer PCR techniques should become a useful diagnostic tool as supplies of antigen for specific antibody detection are limited. The typical facial appearance of 'slapped cheeks' is more commonly seen in children (**7**). The contagious nature of the illness, which is transmitted to about 50% of susceptible contacts (presumably by aerosol), is reflected in its alternative title of erythema infectiosum.

In an individual patient the differential diagnosis is wide and includes enteroviral infections (which often involve palms/soles or mucosal membranes), glandular fever, CMV, HIV seroconversion illness, atypical scarlet fever or attenuated measles and drug rashes. The duration of illness and lack of high fever at onset make exanthema subitum (roseola infantum, human herpes virus 6) less likely. If the patients had visited an endemic area, rickettsial illnesses, such as Rocky Mountain spotted fever, would have been considered. Arbovirus infections, such as dengue, can produce a similar picture in non-immune travellers.

3   Sequelae are more common in adults, although the first patient recovered uneventfully once his fever had settled (**8**). Parvovirus B19 infection should be excluded in adults with unexplained arthritis. The second patient had a more prolonged convalescence, with persistent adenopathy 3 weeks later and a tendency for the rash to recur after exercise. Transient marrow depression is common and these patients had short-lived falls in haemoglobin – from 16.5 to 12.2 g/dl in the first patient and from 14.4 to 12.9 g/dl in the second. Marrow aplasia is more important in patients with pre-existing haemopoietic disorders and those with HIV infection, and is responsible for the majority of episodes of aplastic crisis in patients with sickle cell disease and other haemolytic anaemias.

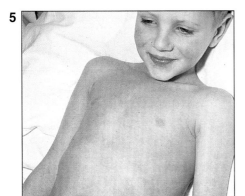

5 Typical rubella rash in a child.

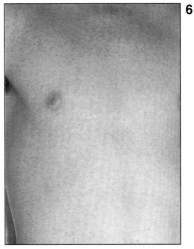

6 The rash of rubella may have a papular component.

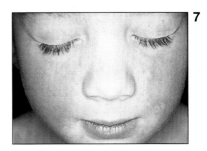

7 Typical appearance of parvovirus B19 infection in a child (slapped cheek).

8 Temperature chart of first patient.

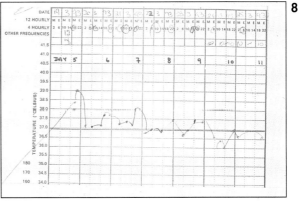

Case 32

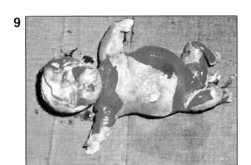

9 Hydrops fetalis caused by parvovirus B19.

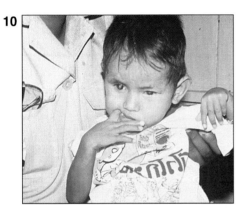

10 Congenital rubella syndrome – a Thai boy with microcephaly, cataracts and deafness.

4 Intrauterine infection with parvovirus B19 has been associated with hydrops fetalis (**9**) and intrauterine death in up to 10–20% of maternal infections (often asymptomatic), the main risk period being the first half of pregnancy. The risk of congenital malformation is minimal if the pregnancy proceeds and is not an indication for termination of pregnancy. There is no vaccine. Because so many infections can mimic rubella, a past history of clinically diagnosed German measles does not rule out acute rubella. Serological diagnosis of the index case is important if he or she has been in contact with a pregnant woman.

The consequences of rubella in pregnancy are well known, with a 90% chance of features of the congenital rubella syndrome in infants of mothers infected during the first ten weeks of pregnancy, falling to less than 20% by 16 weeks (**10**). Infection during this risk period constitutes medical grounds for termination of pregnancy if desired by the mother. The serological status of any pregnant woman in contact with a possible case of rubella for up to 7 days before or 4 days after onset of a rash should be determined. Post-exposure prophylaxis with pooled human normal immunoglobulin does not protect susceptible contacts from infection but may limit clinical symptoms and possibly reduce risk of transmission to the fetus. Active vaccination is contraindicated during pregnancy because the vaccine contains a live attenuated virus, but the mother should be immunised after delivery and seroconversion to vaccine confirmed.

Index

Page numbers in **bold** refer to illustrations